OWN YOUR EATING

THE DEFINITIVE GUIDE
TO FLEXIBLE EATING

JASON ACKERMAN & JAMES MCDERMOTT

Own Your Eating: The Definitive Guide To Flexible Eating

Copyright © 2017 by Jason Ackerman & James McDermott

Editors:
Joanna Toman
Roz Lytle
Patrick Regan
Roz Ackerman
Juanita Smart

Cover design and typesetting by Victor Marcos (99designs.com/profiles/victormarcos)

www.merriam-webster.com (1)
http://cfdanville.com/wp-content/uploads/2014/06/TimeEatButter.jpg
Time Magazine

Printed in the United States of America

To order additional copies of this title visit www.OwnYourEating.com

ISBN:
978-0-692-71779-0 (pbk)
978-0-692-84386-4 (e-bk)

"You can get fat eating broccoli and you can get skinny eating donuts."

- JASON ACKERMAN

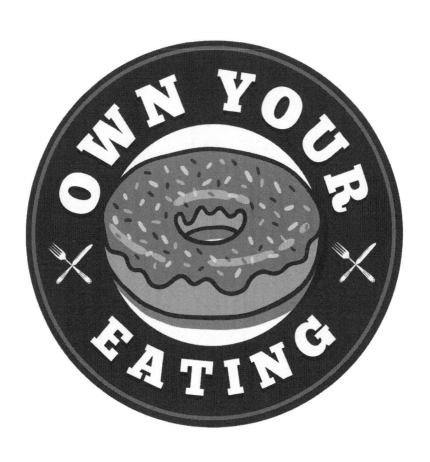

CONTENTS

FOREWORD
by Austin Malleolo

I have known Jason since 2009 when I stumbled into his gym and asked if I could drop in for weekend workouts from time to time. Back then, I would commute to the area to visit my girlfriend, now wife, and it turned into a weekly ritual. The next year, I moved to Albany, NY and for some reason, he hired me as a coach. It was there that I learned so much about CrossFit, coaching, business and met a lot of good people. I would watch Jason run a very successful business, grow a community, teach others and improve the quality of life of everyone that he came into contact with. I also learned firsthand that he was certifiably crazy, passionate, and relentless – these and many other character attributes are what make him so great and unique at what he does.

I often look back and ask myself: *why was he so good?* If you look at all the business tactics, financials, etc. you may in fact be underwhelmed. But, if you take a macro view of what he does – it's simple. He takes the time to care. He would sit in his office in Albany and talk to people either via text, Facebook, face-to-face, or by phone and harass them. He would go out of his way to make people feel like they mattered and he was tireless at proving that fact to them. That is a very rare trait in this world and he embodies it in all that he does. It also showed me what I needed to do to make a difference in other people's lives.

But, the most important lesson I learned from this man was when I told him that I was going to leave Albany CrossFit. I had accepted a coaching job at Reebok CrossFit One; I was so afraid to tell him. I did not want to let Jason down or upset him – he already had done so much for me. When I finally mustered up the courage, his response is one that has shaped how I manage, lead and handle relationships in my life. He simply said that he was happy for me, and that I would be an idiot not to take the opportunity. Of course he was sad to see me leave and said that I would be missed at the gym, but he would never and could never hold me back from an opportunity. His optimism and honest happiness for me as a person was so infectious that it made me feel more confident and proud to have called him a mentor and friend.

Since then Jason and I have drifted apart and back together again working on the CrossFit Seminar Staff. I have seen him do amazing things from afar in business and in life. He calls me for advice at times and I'm reminded of the impact he's had on my life. He reminds me of how amazing life is and how rare it is to find someone as humble and passionate as Jason.

Now, he's co-written a book, about a topic that I am very passionate about myself – nutrition. Proper nutrition forever changed my life and he has set out on a path to help others in their journey to changing theirs. His goal is to spread the word on what has worked for him and has shared it with anyone who will listen. If you are on any of the social media outlets, you've probably seen his posts. He is relentless in his pursuit, a mindset we all can take and apply to our own lives if we want to be successful.

These pages will be filled with knowledge, experience and passion. You will learn about nutrition and how to implement it into your lifestyle. I also urge you to read between the lines – to discover how this book came to be and why this topic is so important to Jason.

I urge you to ask yourself, how did he garner this skill set and knowledge to help so many people? If you ask yourself this question and you are honest with your own answers, you will get more than you can imagine from this book.

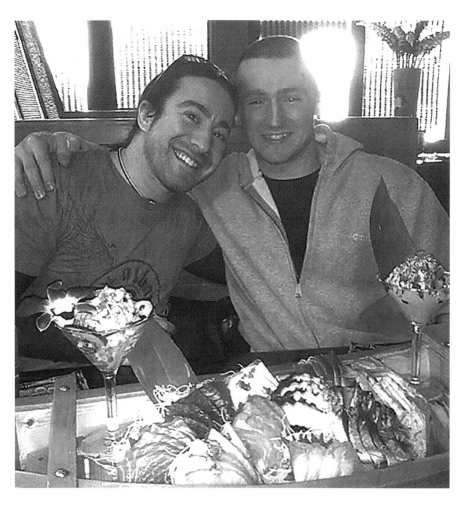

CHAPTER 1

OWN YOUR EATING

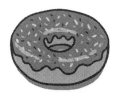

Think back to when you were a kid and try to recall your most favorite food to eat – we all have one. Something that you loved so dearly that the mere thought of it had you frothing at the mouth and crippled with hunger pangs until that craving was satisfied. Mine was the cheesiest, gooiest, most mouthwatering bowl of macaroni and cheese. In fact, it's still my favorite food to this day. But, I'm not just talking about any old melty pasta dish – I'm talking about the one and only Kraft Mac & Cheese. Just one whiff of that cheesy goodness or a glimpse of that blue ninety-nine cent box and I'm immediately transported back to my childhood when my mom would whip me up the biggest bowl with extra love and care.

I'm sure your favorite food brings you that wave of nostalgia too. Sadly, though, there was a brief time in my life where enjoying some Mac & Cheese no longer brought back fond memories. It became synonymous with a "cheat day." Instead of bringing me warm & fuzzy feelings of comfort and joy, my beloved meal would leave me feeling immensely guilty and ashamed.

I know I don't speak alone here when I tell you that deprivation **IS** awful, both mentally and physically. Suppressing your desire to have your favorite treat because it is somehow "bad" is no way to live your life.

I'm overjoyed to tell you it **DOESN'T** have to be this way ever again. You can eat the foods you love while fueling your body properly and keeping your nutrition on point. Your taste buds and mind will thank you endlessly for this. That is what makes the Flexible Eating lifestyle so unique – by design it will nourish the body and make you feel **HAPPY** about what you are eating and help you create the balance your body craves.

This book will teach you how to live a lifestyle that is realistic and sustainable in our modern world. To do that we will utilize a number of tools within the text such as inspirational stories where you can learn from the experiences of others who have been where you are now, equations and diagrams that will help you calculate how much food you would ideally eat each day, and chapter assessments (beginning after Chapter 3). Self-critical analysis is a super important part of any one person's individual growth. Use these assessments to take pause at the end of each chapter and reflect inward on yourself. The more you apply the knowledge within this book to yourself, take ownership of your current missteps, and take action toward correcting them the better. Through all of that you will learn how to be happy about the things you eat, gain the ability to go to bed eager to wake up the next morning and achieve your goals one meal at a time, and most importantly you will learn how to...

OWN YOUR EATING!!

CHAPTER 2

FLEXIBLE EATING MINDS

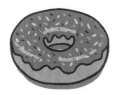

JASON'S STORY

Growing up in the 80's, I lived a lifestyle of your typical skinny kid. My parents had concrete boundaries on eating snack foods, and since my mother was a great cook, we rarely ate out at restaurants. There was always a big emphasis on homemade meals made from whole foods. If you were hungry you ate, if you were full you stopped. I learned to keep things simple and reasonable from my mother, but on the other hand, I often observed that my father and stepmother were very into "fad diets," but never encouraged me to try them.

I never really thought about my body weight until I started my four-year journey into middle school wrestling. I competed in the 91 lbs. weight class, at first, which was easy to maintain. Eventually during my sophomore year, I had to keep an eye on the scale and what I ate.

It's important to understand that in those days there was no such thing as nutrition coaching. No one was available to give proper guidance and whatever advice I received came mainly from my teammates. "Go home and eat ice for dinner and have some Advil for dessert" was the prescription for cutting weight before a big meet. My parents didn't know any better; they just thought it was what I needed to do to participate in the sport.

My junior year was definitely the most stressful when it came to cutting weight and usually meant starving myself until I reached my goal weight. It was during this time that I started to develop binge-eating habits that affected me for years to follow. I continued the cut weight / wrestle / binge cycle all throughout high school where I competed in the 130 lbs. weight class. I finally decided to stop my senior year – enough was enough.

I gave up wrestling the summer after high school and set my eyes on being a fit and healthy person – as an added bonus, bodybuilding became a new pursuit. It was during this time that I found not only a love for weight training, but helping others achieve their goals as well. A typical day for me included interning at the gym for a couple hours which was followed by my own workout.

It was at Club Fit where I met my old friend Mike Longo who helped me pursue bodybuilding a little more seriously. After buckling down on my training and under the guidance of Mike, I decided to do my first official bodybuilding show. I took second place in the teen division weighing 115 lbs. and later on that summer I took first place at my second show.

I was beginning to understand more about nutrition and how to be disciplined with my diet. I mainly ate a diet of egg whites, oatmeal, chicken, rice, broccoli, and sweet potatoes. Although I tried to resist them, the old routines were still there and I would often resort to under eating while training hard for shows. After the shows, the restrictiveness of my diet would catch up with me and I would go nuts binge eating entire boxes of cinnamon graham crackers and other sweet foods to satisfy my urges.

These habits continued to haunt me throughout college. I was stuck in a vicious diet cycle of cutting weight before a show and then easily gaining back 30 lbs. after binging and eating carelessly almost in rebellion.

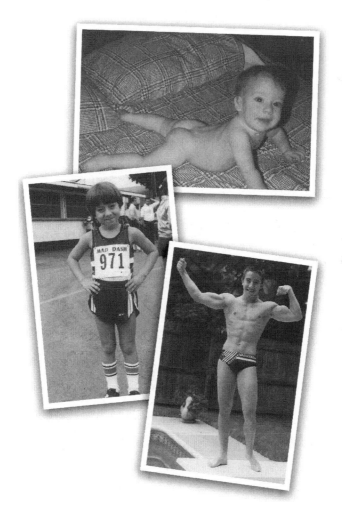

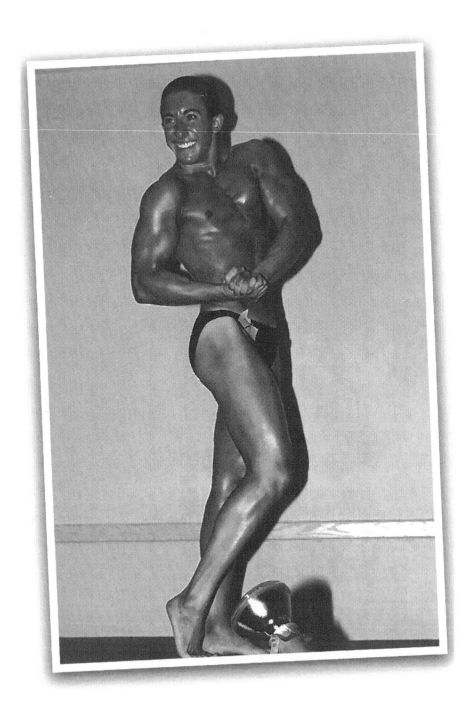

Post college, I found myself living with my girlfriend at the time, doing some light weight training, a lot of yoga, and dabbling in vegetarianism. She and I were just trying to do what we thought was necessary to be healthy people. After adopting two Pugs, I decided to become a full-fledged vegetarian because I couldn't fathom harming animals that were like my dogs – I had a lot of love for them.

Unfortunately, like many vegetarians out there, I ate a very restrictive diet lacking of all things a variety of vegetables. There was absolutely no quality or quantity control – provided there was no meat, everything else was fair game.

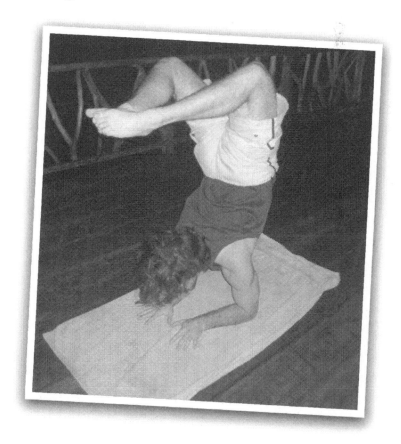

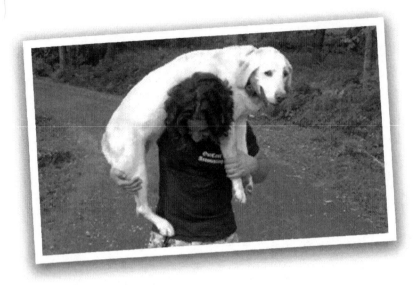

In 2007, I found CrossFit and with it, new revelations about my own personal nutrition.

Much to my surprise I quickly learned that my body could not handle the intense exercise regime. The sheer volume of work done in CrossFit was too much for my vegetarian lifestyle and a change needed to be made.

I attended the CrossFit Level 1 certification with the founder Greg Glassman. It was an incredible experience and I learned a lot that would shape the course of my life over the next decade. Because of what I learned there I started eating meat again to better fuel my body for workouts. What I found through Paleo was a very low carbohydrate mentality. It was all about eating a lot of meat, the glorification of bacon and the vilification of foods like grains. This was a stark contrast to everything I had previously been doing.

Counting macronutrients was definitely not a concern. The Paleo diet was all about the quality of the foods being consumed, but that too had its pitfalls. Soon came justifications for eating anything that was considered *"Paleo"* – even baked treats. Paleo "challenges" were all the rage in those days; which led to a lot of 30-day restrictive diets followed by heavy binge eating on Day 31.

I soon realized that I needed more structure to improve my CrossFit performance and recover from intense workouts. Pairing the quality aspects of Paleo with the quantity methods of the Zone diet seemed like the best idea... However, it was anything but a sustainable lifestyle.

Sure, I developed some good habits such as meal prepping and traveling with food packed in Tupperware, but it wasn't easy. In the quest for virtuosity, I even became "that guy" at the party who wouldn't eat certain things or brought his own meals.

And still, the cycle of diet / binge / diet / binge continued to repeat itself for a few years. I thought I was in great shape! I thought I had the body that I had always wanted! I was wrong on both counts.

Discovering Flexible Eating changed my entire outlook on nutrition and living a healthy lifestyle. Within the first year of practicing this method, I went from weighing 170 lbs. and eating 1,900 calories per day to weighing **140 lbs.** eating **3,000 calories** per day.

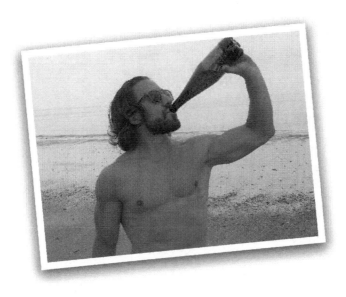

I live a lifestyle that is guilt free, enjoyable, sustainable, and most importantly healthy for both the body and the mind. I no longer restrict my food intake and basically operate under the notion of *"don't eat like an asshole."*

Flexible Eating has also changed my relationship with food to one that is both enjoyable and sensible. I know that this method can change the lives of countless people out there and I hope it does for you what it did for me.

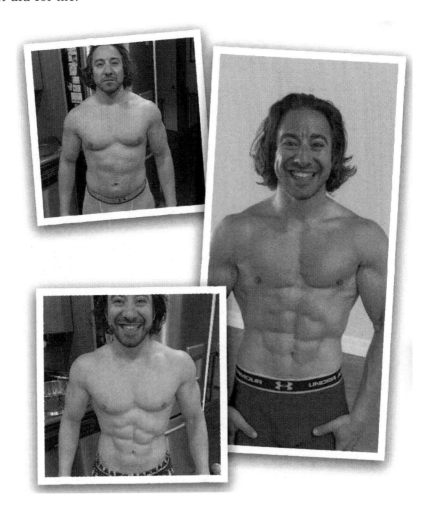

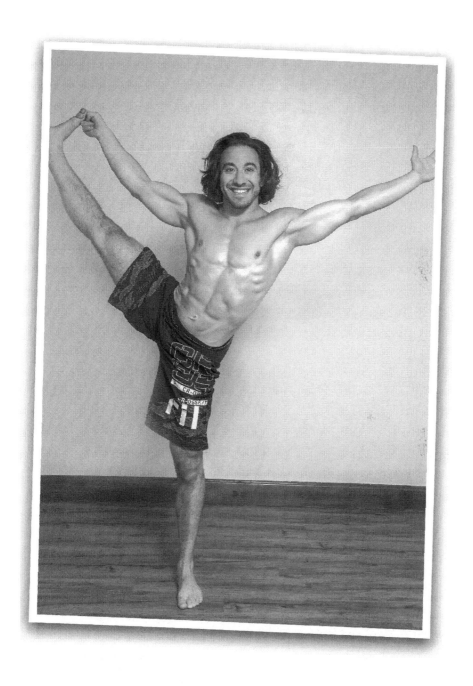

A FLEXIBLE FRIENDSHIP

The peace of mind and confidence that Flexible Eating has provided me with has been unbelievable. Never before would I have thought that it would be possible to eat the foods I love **AND** have a healthy body. In fact, I'm so proud of my physique that you can almost always find me these days shirtless in a photo or video all over social media. You may be thinking that I must just be a vain person, but I assure you I'm not. You certainly wouldn't have seen me so exposed back when I was 190 lbs. with a body that most would have said looked pretty good. So, what's different now? I am at ease. I am comfortable potentially for the first time in my life with my body and who I am as a person. When I look in the mirror, I just see me, and not something I wish was better.

Flexible Eating made me feel empowered as a human being and with that I want to help others feel the same way. That quite simply has always been my mission in life – to help people be better. Throughout the text you will read stories about some of the people I have helped through nutrition. This is not to toot my own horn, but to inspire you. To show you that you're not alone with the dietary struggles you face and that it is indeed possible to change and obtain the lifestyle you want.

The first story, apart from my own, is about *Own Your Eating*'s co-author James McDermott. James is an extremely talented individual, whom I first met back in the summer of 2011, when he came to work as an intern at Albany CrossFit. Those of you that know me well are aware that I just do not have the attention span or patience to sit down and write a whole book – heck I might even be a little lazy when it comes to "paperwork." James, on the other hand, is quite skilled at this kind of thing.

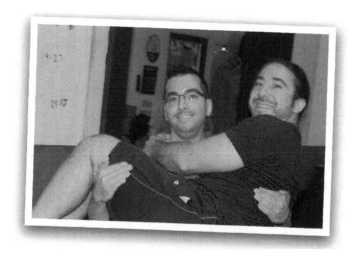

During our time working together at Albany CrossFit, he was always on top of anything computer related whether it be the gym's programming, updating the website, writing articles for the blog, or even typing up his notes from a weightlifting seminar that would one day become the basis for his first book on weightlifting co-written with National Champion Jon North titled The Dark Orchestra. I had known for a little while that I wanted to write a book, but had no idea on where or how to start such a project. After reading The Dark Orchestra I knew I needed to contact James. It has been absolutely wonderful to reconnect through working on this project and refreshing to hear that he has used the knowledge gained to help his own clients and gym. There's no doubt in my mind that you can learn a thing or two from him and his story.

JAMES' STORY

Growing up I was fortunate to have two parents – James and Martha – who provided my sister Anjelica and I with everything our hearts desired. My father was a hardworking, blue collar, Irish man who did all he could to put food on his family's table; there were no problems if it made us happy and tasted good. He was an expert at making bacon and egg breakfast sandwiches in the morning and our summers were filled swimming in our pool and eating hotdogs 'n' hamburgers he cooked on the grill.

We lived in very close proximity to the rest of the family with our house right between my Grandmother Marta's house and my Aunt Lulu's home. Along with my mother, they were always concerned with whether us kids were eating *enough* food and they seemingly never stopped cooking from day to day. Grandma was a master chef who would often make traditional Puerto Rican dishes such as Arroz Con Gandules (rice with pigeon peas), Pernil (pork shoulder), Arroz Con Dulces (rice pudding), and Pasteles (traditional Christmas pastry wrap filled with plantains, meat, and an assortment of vegetables). When you went to Grandma's house, there was no way you were leaving without being served a meal as nothing brought her more joy than to fill the bellies of her grandchildren.

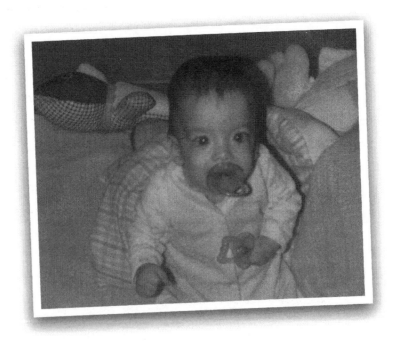

Looking back on it now, I was definitely very well fed, but the issue was that there were **no boundaries** set in regards to food. It was not uncommon for me to eat a meal made by my mother and then run next door to Grandma's for another one. A meal was also always followed with sweet treats – something there was never a shortage of in any household. My mother would bake (almost daily) an assortment of cakes and cookies to have after dinner. If we finished a sheet of delicious chocolate chip cookies, she would make more upon request because it made us happy. Our house was also never short on candies, donuts, soda, and sugary cereals. Often, I would sit in front of the T.V. watching cartoons while shovelling handfuls of Cocoa Puffs straight from the box and into my mouth.

Aside from having bountiful amounts of food provided for me, I was also an *extremely* finicky eater as a child. I enjoyed eating meat

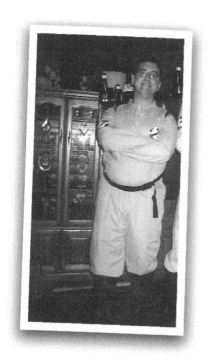

dishes, but hated vegetables to the point where there are many that I have only recently eaten for the first time only as an adult in my mid-twenties such as asparagus, kale, and eggplant. Those peas in Arroz con Gandules? Yeah, I would pick them out and just eat the rice. I would refuse to eat Meatloaf, but would eat Meatballs (same ingredients, but different shape because the shapes of food were important at the time!).

At the very apex of my pickiness, the daily meals were reduced down to: Chef Boyardee's Beefaroni, Lay's Potato Chips dipped in Bumble

Bee's Solid White Tuna Fish mixed with Hellmann's Mayo (it had to be these brands or I wouldn't eat), and plain white bread with butter.

These were the staple foods that made up the bulk of my diet. The only other foods I occasionally would chow down on were chicken, mashed potatoes, pizza, and the aforementioned hamburgers, hotdogs, oh, and plenty of sweets. From age 7 and into my teen years, I could get away with these eating habits. I was very active, playing outside for most of the day, swimming in the pool and participating on youth baseball – I was always a pretty skinny kid.

However, that dynamic changed when my father passed away from a heart attack. He was the one who would push me to get out of the house, or to play sports and with him gone I lost my motivation. After that, instead of running around outside exploring the world, I chose to stay inside exploring a virtual one in video games.

I spent entire summers locked away in my room, and on a typical day, I would wake up at 5:00pm *(nope, that's not a typo!)* in the afternoon after staying up all night and into the early morning playing an online video game called Unreal Tournament 2003. For my first meal, I ate a family sized DeGiorno pizza and then started plugging away at the game. At some point in the evening, I would make myself a couple of Tuna Fish sandwiches to eat along with a bag of Lay's potato chips. My desk was littered with fun sized M&M and baby Snickers bar wrappers and the floor with vanilla Coke cans – I usually finished an entire case in one night. I would go to bed at 7:00am and repeat the cycle the next day.

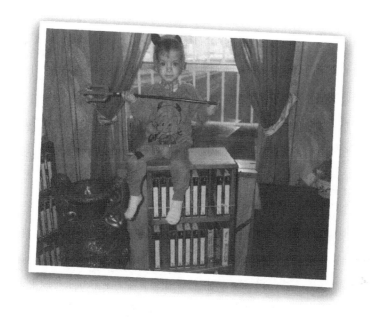

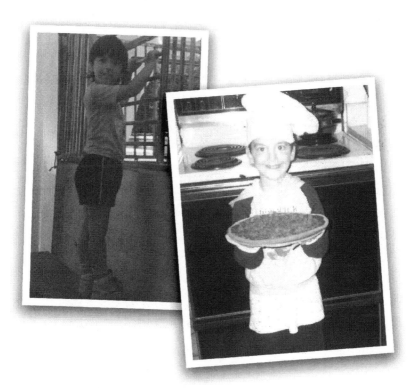

By my sophomore year in high school, I was just over 200 lbs. at 5'5 and in poor health. I had no muscle, strength, or cardiovascular endurance; I could barely walk up the stairs at school without becoming exhausted and winded – I also spent a fair amount of time in and out of the hospital with gastrointestinal issues. The moment that would spark a change for me and shape the rest of my life came one day after a gym class, that I barely participated in. As I walked down the hallway with my gym teacher, Mr. Rapp. He asked me if I ever planned to take my physical fitness seriously and stated "out of all the things you think about, you should think about your health first, nothing else is going to matter if you don't have that." I admit that it took time for those words to make their way through my thick skull, but I eventually took his advice and embarked on a path filled with exercising and dieting.

Flash-forward to the summer after I graduated high school and I was down to 138 lbs. I could run 3 miles in under twenty minutes and played hours upon hours of tennis, instead of video games, with friends. I had established new nutritional habits such as replacing white bread with wheat, ate a lot of chicken 'n' rice, and started carrying around Tupperware filled with my meals. I was absolutely crazy about reading food nutrition labels and avoiding things such as high fructose corn syrup and trans fats. While I was starting to learn about living a "healthy" lifestyle, weight loss to me still meant more running and restricting what I ate. I would eat foods that I perceived to be clean and healthy, but then give in and indulge on the cookies that my mom still made – sometimes I felt bad about it, like I was ruining all of my progress, and other times I felt like it was okay because I earned it. The emotions that came with certain types of foods fluctuated depending on the situation, but that mindset would change when I went to college.

In college, the focus was no longer on losing weight, but to gaining it instead in the form of more muscle. I began to lift weights a little more seriously and soon fell in love with the sport of powerlifting – I wanted to be big and strong! At the time, all the advice I could find to accomplish that goal simply said that I needed to eat **A LOT** of food, ditch running endless miles on the road, and lift heavy things. I did just that and taught myself how to squat, bench press, and deadlift along with eating ridiculous amounts of food. In a year I went from weighing 138 lbs. to 190 lbs. Unfortunately, there was no rhyme or reason to any of what I was doing and as a result, I only became marginally strong and put on a lot of excess body fat.

On top of that, my gastrointestinal problems returned and I ended up relying on antacids to soothe my heartburn. The situation became so bad that a doctor wanted to cut out my gall bladder because of the stones forming within it. I refused the surgery and set out to get my health back on track – eat big, lift big was just not working out. One mistake can often lead into another and I went down some less intelligent paths involving fat burning pills and a large volume of cardio, but I can tell you this: there's no quick 'n' easy route to your goals, only hard work and time.

In 2011, at the end of my sophomore year at SUNY (State University of New York) Cortland, I arrived at Albany CrossFit to fulfill an internship requirement for my Bachelor of Science degree in Kinesiology (the study of human movement). Right off the bat, Jason Ackerman was on my case about my nutrition – and rightfully so – I was doing a terrible job at managing it and was poorly conditioned. With his encouragement, I decided to give the Paleo diet (which was the default CrossFitter way of eating at the time) a shot; if I was going to truly learn about it, I should have some experience following the protocol personally. That summer, I dropped down from 190 lbs. to 150 lbs. Throughout the rest of the year, I dabbled in mixing Paleo and the Zone Diet along with even some intermittent fasting. By the time December rolled around I weighed 143 lbs. and I was completely obsessed with the scale – I always wanted to see that number moving down!

Doing CrossFit and following the Paleo diet I was able to maintain a body weight that fluctuated between 143 lbs. to 155 lbs. for quite some time. However, in October 2013, I had a mini stroke (TIA) and as a result changed the way I was training. After the incident, I had a lot of abnormal trouble breathing in high intensity workouts. I felt like I was slowly being suffocated and it eventually led me to change my training focus to weightlifting. If I couldn't participate in traditional CrossFit training, I might as well work on strength and skills that did not affect me so negatively. By lifting barbells more frequently, I improved my snatch from 115 lbs. to 185 lbs., and my clean and jerk from 165 lbs. to 245 lbs. Many other lifting totals increased as well, but I was mostly concerned with those two lifts as I began to compete in the sport.

This was the first time I was able to put on muscle and strength without ballooning excessively with a lot of extra body fat (although some certainly was gained). I levelled out and competed within the 85 kg (169.422 lbs. to 187 lbs.) weight class typically at a body weight ranging from 177 lbs. to 182 lbs. I was happy with and never really had an issue maintaining this body weight until the 2015 Elmira Spring Open. At around this time, I was in the process of finishing up my first book, The Dark Orchestra.

My diet had definitely slipped and long nights and weekends sitting in front of my laptop definitely interfered with my training and weight management. Most days I was eating one large burrito bowl (triple meat!) at Chipotle and then snacking on Ben & Jerry's ice cream at night.

When I weighed in at the meet, I was over weight for my class and had to lift in the 94 kg (187.002 lbs. to 206.8 lbs.) category instead. I was embarrassed, but it was the kick in the butt I needed to refocus on my health and not just the projects I was working on.

Shortly after, I began ordering pre-made Paleo meals from a local company called MacroNu. I spoke with the owner Chris over the phone and told him my dilemma – I needed meals that tasted good (at the time my cooking skills were lacking), but that were in line with my goals. I find that sticking close to a Paleo-ish way of eating works very well for me. He ensured me that his food was all locally sourced – the meat coming from chicken and cows from down the road – and vegetables grown in their own private garden. He ensured me that they would be able to provide me with multiple meals each day to make sure I was eating more consistently. MacroNu helped me get back on track and trim down for my next competition that summer and I had no problem making weight.

Later that year in November 2015, Jason reached out to me for help with writing this book. So that I could better learn his process, he set me up with my own customized macronutrient numbers based on my goals. I wanted to jump right in, and worked with both Jason and Chris from MacroNu to create custom Paleo meals that were based off of my numbers. Right away I could tell the difference. I thought that eating three meals a day from MacroNu was a lot of food, but I was completely wrong. With these numbers, I was eating so much more protein and felt amazing amounts of energy in my training sessions. I felt stronger, started sleeping a little better, and cravings for snacks started to dwindle away since I was giving my body the correct nutrition it needed to perform.

I looked at the custom meals as Flexible Eating training wheels. They helped me find a balance, plan ahead for a week at a time, and find consistency by eating meals that I enjoyed. Through this whole process I started eating foods (mainly vegetables) that I was still avoiding all these years later. If the meal contained broccoli, kale, spinach, or onions it was no problem – I ate them anyway because hitting the numbers became more important to me than my own aversions towards vegetables. Eventually, when I was ready, I reverted back to ordering regular non-custom meals and practiced filling in the gaps with other foods to meet my macronutrient requirements for the day. This allowed me more freedom to eat other foods that I wanted, but in a sensible amount.

I can honestly say that the whole experience has been life-changing. For the first time, I am able to eat foods with a focus on fueling my body for performance as opposed to pure pleasure. I can eat cookies without inhaling the whole package, but also not feel bad about eating them in the first place. Flexible Eating has changed my entire outlook on nutrition and I'm excited to continue seeing it's benefits not only for myself, but others as well.

After reading our stories, hopefully you realize that Jason and I are normal people just like you. We have both been through some rocky roads in regards to our relationships with food and we're certainly not perfect now as he and I still face the same nutritional obstacles each day that you also experience. Our journeys, along with yours, are set on a path towards the unachievable goal of *perfection*, and while we may never truly get there, it's the time and effort put into your own health and wellbeing that's truly important. We hope that you take the lessons learned within this text to heart and that they help you change your life for the better just as they have ours. Good luck and happy eating!

CHAPTER 3

A VICIOUS CYCLE

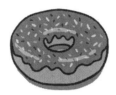

Change
/CHānj/
verb

1. make or become different.
   "an idea to change one's lifestyle"
2. take or use another instead of.
   "she decided to change her diet"

noun

1. the act or instance of making or becoming different.
   "the change from an unhealthy lifestyle to a healthier one"

We have all been there before standing at a crossroads in life filled with the desire to seek out something different for ourselves. You're probably at one right now. I'll bet you're holding this book in your hands with a mindset bent on seeking out a fresh start on your life, a new perspective on how you can be better – a change. Well, I am extremely happy that you are taking serious steps in the direction of achieving your personal goals and honored that I can tag along for the ride.

To be honest with you; the road ahead will not be an easy one, heck it might even be a little scary. But, that's perfectly okay! Anything worth pursuing will come with challenges and I can tell you from personal experience that you are going to do just fine. I plan to give you every resource I have to help guide your success in the simplest most efficient ways possible.

My mission is to make sure you learn a lot! Not only about things such as metabolism, different types of macronutrients, and my methodology, but also a lil' bit about yourself. Those other topics are super important, but **YOU** are the key to your own success. Learning about yourself, more specifically about your eating habits and personal relationships with food, will be a huge part of this way of eating.

Let's start simple. I'll set the stage with a scene that's all too familiar...

It's December 31st – New Year's Eve. New York City is busier than ever as millions gather in droves to watch that world renowned ball take its annual plunge. Whether you are in the Big Apple in person, or watching on T.V., this magical crystal ball has the power to wipe the slate clean. We gaze upon it in wonder, eyes hungry for change and our hearts filled with hope...the countdown begins...

24

10... I want...no...I **NEED** to make a change!

9... This year will be different, I can do this.

8... I've slacked off for far too long.

7... I'm sick and tired of being sick and tired!

6... I need to do this for my health, for me.

5... My success will blow everyone away.

4... I cannot wait to hear what my family and friends say!

3... I'm going to be in the best shape of my life!

2... I promise myself that I will not fall back off the wagon.

1... **TOMORROW**...is Day One...

The countdown ends and a new year begins! You are filled with motivation...and just a little bit of alcohol *(okay, maybe a lot)*. It's time to get started!

The next day, late into the morning you wake up...slightly *(or, heck, maybe even heavily)* hungover. Yet, you have a renewed attitude towards your personal health. You, along with countless others around the world, are about to embark upon the various phases of a sort of master plan to a lifestyle renovation.

- **Phase One:** Purchase a membership to a now overcrowded gym.
- **Phase Two:** Purge your cupboards and refrigerator until every last morsel of the food you once enjoyed is gone.
- **Phase Three:** Now that all the junk food is in the trash you need to restock the fridge. Pack it full of all the raw veggies and poached chicken that you now plan to eat exclusively for the rest of your life (or at least for 30 days).
- **Phase Four:** Boy, shopping is exhausting...time to recover at Applebee's with a few friends and order off the "fit 'n' healthy" part of the menu because that's the only section you're allowed to eat from now, right?

Flash-forward one week in and everything is going so well! You've lost a few pounds, clothing is fitting a little better, and you like what you see in your full-length mirror. You keep surfing this wave of positivity right into week two. Unfortunately, by its end the waters have become a little less inviting. Something feels just...*off*...not like it did during those first few days... but you can't quite put your finger on it...

Then you realize: this new **YOU** is not fitting in well with the rest of *real life*. At social gatherings you start to feel a little out of place and maybe even guilty for having that drink with a friend, or a bite of that dish you always *used* to order at your favorite restaurant. Speaking of your friends, they support you but ultimately do not understand why you're following the diet of a rabbit. Though their comments bear no malice – you resent having to explain yourself to everyone under the sun!

Enter week three and that #motivationalmonday vibe you have been feeling is weakening. You still squeeze workouts in here and there, but you find yourself making justifications (to yourself and others) on why it is okay for you to have that treat. You say it's because of how *"good"* you have been lately – you've earned it at the gym. At first these treats are isolated incidents. Then these scenarios start to play out almost daily. There's the Snickers bar or two at lunch and then full on binge on the weekend.

Week four – a pivotal crossroads. The scale no longer greets you with a smile and a surprise of a lower weight every morning. Instead, a constant battle is being waged between the devil on your left shoulder beckoning you to indulge your cravings – and the angel on your right reminding you of the promises you made to yourself at the beginning of the year.

Your eyes wander around the gym and you notice it's not as crowded as it used to be. Some of those machines are empty now like many of the New Year's Resolutions that filled them in the first place. That path to a new lifestyle – a new and improved you has been abandoned – the resolution doomed from the very moment it was created. Back to the drawing board – maybe, next year will be different...right?

WRONG.

But, what you need to realize is that this cycle doesn't need to keep repeating itself; there is indeed a better way. Throughout this book you're going to learn a lot of science, strategies, and methods that combine to form my holistic approach towards eating, and obtaining the personal lifestyle you desire. However, before we can go into great detail about all of that, we need to begin a serious discussion.

We need to talk about your personal relationship with food.

Whether you realize it or not, you have a relationship with food, and with the way that you eat. It is a special bond that is, to some extent, no different and just as powerful as the one you share with your friends and family.

Let's learn a little about that relationship and your habits right now. Grab a pen and a piece of paper!

1   Take a look in your fridge and cabinets and rate your pantry on a scale of **(1)** You keep Doritos in business... to: **(5)** Your diet is so fresh and clean you eat baby carrots as a movie theater snack!

RATE

2   How do you feel about the types of foods you keep handy?

CHAPTER 4

A WORD ON METABOLISM

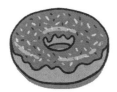

Remember my goal is not only to teach you about my nutritional methods, but a bit about yourself as well. Maybe your story is like mine, or James'. Or, maybe your story is a little different than the New Year's scenario depicted earlier – that's cool – we have all *been there* at one time or another. The key to success is to figure out **WHY** it never worked and what you can do to change and live a happy and sustainable lifestyle that caters to your goals.

If you feel you are someone who has a grip on their personal relationship with food and just want to dive right into the meat and potatoes of how to get started, then feel free to skip ahead to *Chapter 9 - Hit Your Numbers*, where we'll teach you how to calculate your personal macronutrient numbers. For the rest of you, we have much to learn, let's discuss a common topic amongst those looking to gain or lose weight: **Metabolism.**

I see it all the time: "10 ways to boost your metabolism" or "set your metabolism on fire to get shredded!" I'm sure there are some tips in articles such as these that may prove helpful, but what I have found to be the cornerstone to altering your metabolism is **consistency**. Instead of fixating on 10 different ways to improve your metabolism and doing so only half-heartedly, choose to focus on consistency alone. If you are consistent with hitting your numbers above all else, then I can promise you, you will reignite and boost your metabolism.

So what the heck is metabolism? Straight from the dictionary: "the chemical processes by which a plant or an animal uses food, water, etc., to grow and heal and to make energy." (1) Typically, when someone is talking about their "metabolism," what they are actually referring to is their resting metabolic rate (RMR). Your RMR is the number of calories your body needs to sustain all of its important operations necessary to live such as:

- Maintaining your body temperature.
- Pumping blood throughout vessels to organ and tissues.
- Consuming and transporting oxygen.
- Delivering nutrients in and out of cells.

These functions are, obviously, vital and occur naturally when you are at rest i.e. sitting and reading this book right now.

How does all of this affect your body weight, you ask? Well, your body composition (how much muscle tissue you carry) plays a huge role in the efficiency of your metabolism. At rest (just chillin'), someone who has a greater amount of muscle mass will burn more calories sustaining that tissue than someone of the exact same weight who is sedentary and has less muscle mass.

We can assume the person who has a sedentary lifestyle naturally has more body fat. Fat is a tissue that is not as "metabolic" as muscle meaning that at rest it takes much less energy to maintain. That makes perfect sense because fat is meant to be stored energy. Our body holds onto fat in-case of a crisis situation like starvation…or a five mile run. On the flipside, strong, shapely muscle tissue not only takes more effort to build, but the body needs to do more work to keep it. That means supplying muscles with nutrients to continue building and repairing them – a process that will require energy (burning calories) because work in the body has a price.

Our metabolisms aren't inherently or unchangeably slow or fast, but they are aspects of ourselves which respond to cues and care. Your metabolism is only slow if you make it that way.

It is not a static tragic characteristic we have to learn to work around like a big nose or an affinity towards Nickelback. Some of us just have physiology that is currently running very inefficiently because of our own **personal habits** coupled with adhering to what is considered **conventional wisdom**.

METABOLIC FIRE

To paint this picture in a different light let's imagine we're building a fire together and draw some parallels between the materials you would need and your body; then we will put it all together and discuss how your metabolism works in a similar way.

- First, the Home-Depot-Approved fire pit (your body) needs to be set up. This is what controls the fire (your metabolism).
- Next you lay down the coals for a foundation. This is our "body fat" – the slow burning energy.
- On top of the coals pile on a bunch of logs or in this regard our "muscles."

- Also insert little things such as branches or rolled up newspaper (food).
- Every fire needs oxygen (exercise or physical activity) to thrive!
- Finally, when all of that is in the pit...you spray on some lighter fluid, throw in the match, and watch the flames take hold, or in other words, the motivation to get started.

Now, if we had only coals in the pit we would have a very poor fire. Yes, the coal is going to burn for a long period of time, but it cannot take us to the next level if we are trying to build a big fire. We need to add more robust materials into the pit that will burn up more rapidly and produce the raging monster of a fire we want. This is where the logs – our muscles – come into play. With more of them in the pit the fire grows, heat intensifies and more energy is produced. Or in the case of a human being, more calories are burned both at rest and during activity.

The more muscle you build (or logs you add to the pit), the greater the fire becomes.

While you are there roasting marshmallows and making s'mores you need to keep **FEEDING** the fire or you will lose it. The beauty is that this fire is nourished by any number of things (just like your body is). You add more logs, yes, but you also get the same result of a thriving fire by throwing in some branches and rolled up newspaper – i.e. you need to eat food. The amount needs to be just right, if you throw in too much, you might just smother the fire – if you put in too little it will be weak and eat away too much at the logs.

So in reality...you are not overweight because your metabolism is slow. You are overweight because of how you are managing your metabolic fire. You need to establish better eating habits that allow you to *eat the right amount of food consistently*.

So, we have our fuel, heat is being produced, but one more thing is necessary to truly ignite a fire – oxygen (exercise). You need to exercise –

more specifically weight train to promote building muscles (and not spending countless hours on the treadmill). Living a sedentary lifestyle coupled with erratic eating is a guaranteed way to promote excess body fat and mess with your body's physiology. You need to take action, to light the match, and go for it. Without the motivation to change we can have nothing!

> *** Important side note:** We **ALL** need muscle mass to help our metabolism function efficiently. Ladies, you will not become "bulky" if you weight train. Your body simply does not have the necessary amount of testosterone for that to happen. It is a common misconception that training with weights will produce that result.

Take a break from reading and give yourself a moment or two to digest what you just read. Use this time to think about your eating habits and current relationship with food.

3   What are three things you feel you are doing correctly in your relationship with food?

(1) ....

....

....

(2) ....

....

....

(3) ....

....

....

4   What are three areas you feel you could improve upon?

(1) ....

....

....

(2) ....

....

....

(3) ....

....

....

CHAPTER 5

MARIA'S NOT SCARED ANYMORE!

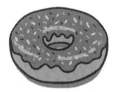

I first met Jason eight years ago at Albany CrossFit. Although he is someone that I deeply respect and admire, I have to admit I had some reservations about Flexible Eating. We had talked about it a few times, but I just could not buy into the concept. I was coming from a figure athlete – bodybuilding – background and had my meal plan hanging from the fridge and followed it meticulously every single day. It was downright scary to think about eating the number of carbs Jason recommended.

Jason was definitely relentless, and continually promised me that I would love Flexible Eating. He eventually convinced me to do the right thing for my own health and I can honestly say it was the best decision I have ever made – truly life changing. In the end it was his passion, enthusiasm and belief in his methods that sparked me to give it a shot. Jason has always had a knack for knowing when someone is in need of help and I definitely did. I needed to make serious adjustments to my lifestyle and the push he gave me was just the thing to get me out of my comfort zone.

You see my relationship with food had been one that was filled with absolute terror. I suffered from a condition called Orthorexia, where a person is literally afraid to eat foods they do not consider "clean," and because of that I deprived myself of certain foods for years. I would miss social events and even date nights with my husband because I knew I would freak out if the restaurant had bread on the table.

It saddens me to think about how much I have missed out on because of how I viewed food. To make matters even worse, I would restrictively eat for long periods of time and then suddenly go off the rails when I finally gave into temptation. I would binge so badly and then feel horribly guilty afterwards. Mentally, I was defeated by the choices I made during those episodes, but the problem wasn't the foods that I was eating, but instead my outlook on nutrition.

Flexible Eating was just the remedy I needed to enter into a healthier state of mind when it comes to food. I am **SO HAPPY** to be able to say that a lot of the guilt and fear of eating certain types of foods is behind me now for good. Now, when I become a little anxious, and doubts fill my head, I take a moment to regroup. A little positive self-talk can really go a long way and I just tell myself "you know what just do your best!"

I remember during my first week of Flexible Eating ordering a soft serve vanilla ice cream cone with sprinkles and being elated to finally be able to *"have"* this treat, but more importantly not feel like I wanted to binge afterwards. That's because I was satisfied with both the serving and the knowledge that if I wanted that cold creamy treat again the next day **I COULD HAVE IT**! All I had to do was plan it into my day so it fit my macros – what an incredibly freeing feeling.

Flexible Eating has become a concrete part of my life now. It has given me something I never thought would be possible – control over my dietary habits. Years ago, I would have thought you were crazy if you told me that I would be eating rice every night and ice cream on the weekends and still have the body I want. Now, everything is so different. I can go to an office party and not have anxiety about the cake because I have trust in myself. I can go out on a date night with my husband, eat a delicious hamburger, and focus on him and our conversation instead of food.

Bread on the table? No big deal!

The whole process has me feeling so full of energy and life. I was suffering before Jason came to the rescue with Flexible Eating, and after years of dieting, I have finally learned to not be afraid of food. Eating should be simple. What you put in your mouth shouldn't affect you the way it was affecting me on a psychological level. This is honestly the first time in my life I'm healthy both physically and mentally. When I look in the mirror I am proud of what I see and when I think about all the carbs I eat now I just smile – my life is truly changed and I am forever grateful.

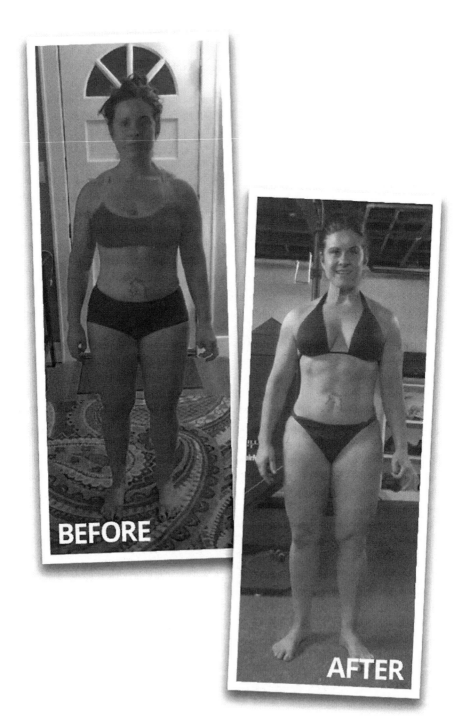

CHAPTER 6

FLEXIBLE EATING, DEFINED

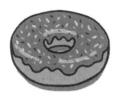

You and I are a team now! A dynamic duo (wearing stretchy underpants and capes) embarking on a mission to dive into the depths of your relationship with food. All you have to do is be as honest as is (super) humanly possible. Exposing hidden truths, that you might not have even known existed can be scary, but together we can use this knowledge to build better, healthier habits.

Our relationship with food is a huge part of our lives, yet we seldom realize just how integral and influential it is. When you're upset, stressed out, or just having a bad day – who is there to take the edge off? A hot, gooey, bowl of mac & cheese! Those creamy golden noodles only have soul-soothing on their mind! When you need a shoulder to cry on after a tough breakup, where do you turn? Ben & Jerry are always there to comfort you with a pint (or two) pints of Phish Food.

But food, and our relationship with it, does not only come into play during Eeyore-like moments – it's usually right there during times of celebration as well. Maybe it's your birthday, an anniversary, or when you start that new job! Basically, for better or for worse, food is the one constant; it is always there. And it always *will* be there, so it's important that you take a step back and examine whether food plays a toxic, or otherwise negative role in your life. Once we have identified whether there is a problem or not we can work towards turning that relationship into a productive (even fun!) one.

So, now here we are…Our hearts are in the right place and we are armed with the knowledge that we *can* ultimately fix a dysfunctional relationship with food, and we *can* combat the mythical "slow metabolism." We know the steps to accomplish this are:

- Using consistency to correct our metabolism.
- Learning about and healing our personal relationship with food.
- Establishing new and sustainable habits.
- Loading our iPods with the Dave Mathews Band anthology *(trust me on this…)*

All with a little help from our new friend; **FLEXIBLE EATING.**

FLEXIBLE EATING DEFINED

Pardon me, I'm about to get a little sciencey...

Flexible Eating is the consumption of a specific amount (usually measured in grams) of macronutrients, the number of which is determined by the required number of calories your body needs to support physical activity or exercise, not excess body fat. It is a method that is born from a place of logic and individualized evaluations. The amount, and macronutrient breakdown of that amount of food that a person needs to eat is based on their own activity level and goals.

The personalized nature of this program, along with its empirically derived numbers, is what allows for the ignition of the metabolism, and the sustainability of it is what allows for the establishment of a healthier relationship with food.

> *Woah, that was intense...I may have blacked out there for a moment explaining that, but all joking aside that is what Flexible Eating is. Let's dig deeper into WHY I think it's such an awesome thing that can help you.*

THE BENEFITS

Throughout my life, I can honestly say I have probably done it all trying to find that magic cure-all for weight loss. Regardless of the nutritional method I was practicing, one aspect was always present – the constant cycles of binge eating and then working to cut weight – it all started to blur together.

Thankfully, though, I can finally say that I **no longer** have that problem since I've adapted to Flexible Eating. It's the only method that allows me to meet my goals and get the results I'm looking for, and is actually sustainable in real, everyday life. All the other diets I have tried have been cycles of restrictions and rewards. I've never been able to follow them long-term since they lacked a clear connection between my goals and my lifestyle. That is why I have taken a sharpie to that ugly word (diet) and eliminated it from my vocabulary and my mindset; I suggest you do the same. Eat flexibly – not only does it sound better, but its more freeing and allows you to live your life and not restrict it.

HERE'S WHY:

1. **Effectiveness:**

   Although quality is still important, *quantity* is the greater determining factor in weight loss or gain. Flexible Eating allows you to eat the exact amount of food you need per day, no more and no less. Because one size does not fit all – your macronutrient numbers are designed for you – your body, your lifestyle. **AND,** there's logic behind it so the guesswork is taken right out from the start. By tracking everything that enters your mouth, you *take control.* Tracking your macros is hands down the most effective way to change your body.

2. **Flexible:**

   Flexible Eating is just that. I keep repeating this because it's one of the most important messages you can take from this book. By focusing on your intake of macronutrients, rather than specific types of foods, you can achieve your goals while enjoying life with everyone else. **You can literally have your cake and eat it too!**

   One of the challenges I have always found with "dieting" is that sometimes- awkward social element that usually goes along with it. There are only so many times you can lug around containers full of rice and chicken before you start getting serious looks. You don't have to be that person. By instead following this program, you can eat flexibly and join in on meals with family and friends, just so long as you keep track of what you're eating.

3. **Sustainable:**

   Since Flexible Eating doesn't restrict you from eating certain foods or your favorite desserts, the "crime and punishment" aspect of most diets is taken away. If you know you're going out with friends for dinner, plan your meals around it for the day. That way there's no guilty feeling if you have that piece of pie for dessert. It gives you a plan to succeed without the pain of sacrifice – which is usually the reason why most diets fail.

Flexible Eating is the first thing that I have been sticking to consistently over a long period of time. From my research and my own personal experience, it kills the "Diet, Binge" cycle that many of us have found ourselves on.

> *It works because it's sustainable. It's sustainable because it caters to your emotional and mental needs (eating the foods you actually want to) as much as it does your physical ones.*

QUANTIFYING NUTRITION

Imagine this, you walk into your gym and your trainer has this written on the board:

BACK SQUATS
PULL-UPS

Your first question will probably be one of "how many sets and reps am I meant to do?" or "how heavy are the back squats?" Basically, you'll want to know all about the quantity – the numbers!

We realize the importance for quantifying aspects of our workouts, but sometimes fail to apply that same mindset towards our nutrition. Chances are you know how much you bench press. You probably know to the second the time of your fastest 5k or your best Fran time if you CrossFit. But, do you know how much protein, carbohydrates, or fat you need to consume to fuel not only your workouts, but your life? Probably not (and you're not alone in that!).

This part of fitness and health is taken for granted. I can tell you from personal experience that you can't out-train a shitty diet and you most certainly need to think about the numbers to get to where you want to go.

MACRONUTRIENTS

Macronutrients, or as we in the biz call them, "macros," are the building blocks and the fuel sources that our bodies use to keep us alive, upright and mobile. Without them, the engine we call our body could not "go" for very long and would eventually keel over. So, it's time now to get familiar with this trio:

- **Protein:** a building block for muscle, that the body can also *convert* to energy to make up for a lack of other macronutrients.
- **Carbohydrates:** a *quick* digesting energy source.
- **Fat:** a *slow* digesting energy source.

After being ingested, these macros provide the body with specific amounts of energy to either build muscle tissue, become stored as fat tissue, or provide fuel to be used during activity. Our primary means of measuring macronutrients is in grams **(g)**. The breakdown is as follows:

- 1g of **Protein** or **Carbohydrates** = 4 Calories.
- 1g of **Fat** = 9 Calories.

CALORIES IN VS. CALORIES OUT

When it comes down to it, calories in vs. calories out is at the foundation of our blueprint, but, as I've mentioned before, it is much more nuanced than this simple, catch phrase. Eating flexibly goes beyond the conventional tenets of eating less to weigh less, and relying solely on the mercy of your scale as a means of judging success.

Don't get me wrong, the scale is still an important tool that we will indeed utilize, but it should only provide an indication that things are going in the right direction. It is certainly not an end all be all. I urge you to avoid the emotional distress that comes with being caught up in the numbers on the scale. A bathroom scale can never explain for the *natural fluctuations* that occur daily. A scale cannot, and does not, take into account water or salt retention, the time of day, or, looking at you, ladies, the time of the month. The scale, for all intents and purposes, is pretty stupid…*literally.*

The number on that machine doesn't and shouldn't define anyone. What should define you is that cholesterol medicine you just kicked to the curb, or the two pant sizes you just dropped, or any other non-numerical triumph you can achieve from nourishing your body properly, with the right quantities of nutrients. What it's really about is finding the energy to not only exercise, but the strength and stamina to push when your workout gets tough. It's about getting a PR for the first time ever and basking in that accomplishment. Any and all of that totally outweighs any number on a silly ole scale.

We would all love to continually see the number on the scale slowly dwindle down to something that puts a smile on our faces. In that ideal world the pounds would melt off you and the results would look like **Figure 6.1**. In reality **Figure 6.2** is more like what you will experience and that's entirely normal. There will indeed be plenty of ups and downs, but with persistence and a growth mindset we can overcome those obstacles.

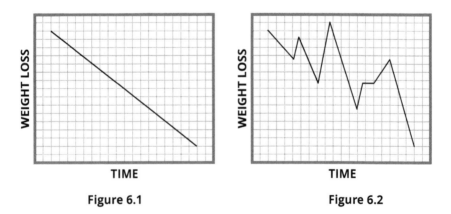

Figure 6.1   Figure 6.2

Take a break from reading and give yourself a moment or two to digest what you just read. Use this time to think about your eating habits and current relationship with food.

5 Thinking back on your answers in the last chapter, what actions will you take to improve in those areas? Try to be as specific and thorough as you can.

CHAPTER 7

BUILDING BLOCKS

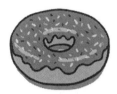

Food can play a powerful psychological role in how we deal with life. We've all had those moments where we question what we just finished shovelling into our mouths. It might have been that seventh piece of pizza, the deep-fried Oreo cookies, or the free refill on that large popcorn at the movies. Everyone's been there at some point and it's moments like that where we should evaluate our emotional relationship with food. When life events happen that trigger these decisions the best thing to do is to write it all down so you can reflect on it later. This system of record and review is a great tool that can help you better understand your relationship with food and why you eat what you eat as well as when you eat it. Let's keep searching for answers together and along the way learn about the inner workings of Flexible Eating and the importance of each macronutrient.

PROTEIN

Protein is by far the most objectively popular macronutrient – from both a cultural and a physiological standpoint. Protein is such a popular source of nourishment that an entire industry is dedicated to it (complete with an endless array of ads selling pretty much the exact same thing). However, "protein" is actually an umbrella term used to refer to a variety of amino acids.

There are three different types of amino acids: **Essential, Semi-Essential** and **Non-Essential.**

- **Essential:** There are eight essential amino acids: isoleucine, methionine, valine, lysine, threonine, phenylalanine, leucine and valine. Now, it is important to note that just because these are called "essential" doesn't mean they are more important than the others. All twenty amino acids are extremely important for various processes within the body, but the essential are the ones we **MUST** consume as part of a balanced diet because they cannot be produced by the body internally.
- **Semi-Essential:** There are two semi-essential acids – Arginine and Histidine. These types of amino acids are needed with advanced age or in situations of physical or mental distress.
- **Non-Essential:** There are ten non-essential amino acids which are readily abundant in the body. To give them their time in the limelight these amino acids are: Alaline, Asparagine, Aspartic Acid, Cysteine, Glutamine, Glutamic Acid, Glycine, Serine, and Tyrosine.

Why are these proteins so important, you may ask? Well, here are just a few of the benefits gained from their consumption:

- **Hypertrophy:** When you exercise you are actually breaking down muscle fibers while you work. Protein is the building block needed to repair those structures damaged by physical activity and to build them up stronger than before.

- **Immune Support:** Protein aids in keeping the immune system functioning by helping to create antibodies (another type of protein) that circulate throughout the bloodstream laying the *Smack Down* on illness.

- **Defends against Catabolism:** Catabolism occurs when an individual is deficient in dietary protein (the essential 8). Your body quite literally starts to "eat" itself when you do not ingest enough of the essential 8 in the form of burning present muscle tissue for energy. No one wants that – especially considering how hard we work for those muscles!

- **Weight Loss:** When you ingest food, the body has to break that food down and process it, meaning it takes energy to burn energy. This process is called the thermic effect of food. Protein requires more effort from the body to breakdown than do carbs or fat. Eating an adequate amount of protein will actually help you lose weight because of the work your body will need to do to digest it. Blend that benefit together with the fact that protein will help you build more muscle, which is more metabolically active at rest, and you have a recipe for success!

These are just a few of the benefits gained from this macro – but for the sake of space (and both mine and your sanity), I'll stop now before we reach a science overload. Instead, let's move forward and talk about the other two macronutrients.

CARBOHYDRATES

Three things need to be addressed immediately:

1. Carbs are not bad for you.
2. A diet too low in carbohydrates is just as damaging as one which is too high in them.
3. Grains (pasta, bread, rice, etc.) **AND** fruits and vegetables are all carbohydrates. It hurts my soul to see the number of people who think that this category only applies to grains.

WHY YOU NEED TO EAT CARBOHYDRATES:

Carbohydrates provide the body with an important – simple sugar – energy source called glucose. This essential fast-acting energy is stored as glycogen in both muscle tissue (for intense activity) and in the liver (for body functions such as central nervous system operation). When you go hard participating in sports such as CrossFit, football, powerlifting, sprinting, or weightlifting the glycogen stored in muscle tissue is converted into glucose, and released into the bloodstream, to support that activity. When those storage centers are depleted, the liver can act as a backup.

What happens though, if you're one of those people who avoid eating carbohydrates because you think they will cause you to gain weight? Well, without carbohydrates to fuel your bodies glycogen depots – protein – is sacrificed for energy and to maintain blood sugar levels through a process called gluconeogenesis. Protein should be used to build big, beautiful muscles and for other important cellular growth and activity. It should not be the body's primary source of energy. Hopefully you are beginning to see the importance of why we need an adequate amount of each macronutrient.

Without balance, you risk spinning your wheels whilst en route towards achieving your goals. When you consume carbohydrates, your body breaks it down and either uses it or stores it in muscle tissues or the liver. But, when you take in more than what your body requires, the excess results in fat storage since there is no room in the other tissues. Make sense? Too much of anything is too much.

Let me emphasize this again one more time – **carbohydrates are a necessary macronutrient**! Love them or hate them; they are a must-have for your body.

FAT

Fat often gets a bad rap and here's why: During the late 1960's and 1970's a series of papers were published on a foundation of faulty research. Unfortunately, people with a lot of money from the food and sugar industry valued their own agenda and making a profit over the health of their customers. The research they funded urged people to limit their fat intake and eat a diet high in protein and carbohydrates. As a result of this prescribed dietary imbalance, the next 30 to 40 years saw millions being affected by illnesses such as heart disease and diabetes.

Heart disease and diabetes became so prevalent because the average person struggles to eat a high protein diet. Most people are so busy that they often forget to eat during the day and when they do have time, they go for whatever the quickest option may be, which is usually things like bagels, bananas, cereals, cookies, donuts, soda and other sugary drinks, pasta, pizza – all the carbs! It certainly can be easy to eat a large number of carbohydrates throughout the day or even in one sitting, but protein takes planning, it takes work.

So what's the problem? The average inactive person who is consuming a large amount of sugar filled carbohydrates, and lacks a balance with the other two macronutrients, is going to begin storing the excess energy as body fat. These carbohydrates also spike a person's insulin, which is a storage hormone within the body, produced by the pancreas, that is tasked with the job of controlling levels of glucose found in the bloodstream. Over time, the body will not be able to produce enough insulin and the unchecked amount of blood glucose can lead to diabetes. The weight gain accompanied by this whole ordeal also certainly contributes to heart disease.

Recently, Time Magazine printed a startlingly different notion, as seen in **Figure 7.1,** on their front cover titled "Eat Butter. Scientists labelled fat the enemy. Why they were wrong." This stands in stark contrast to their publication 30 years earlier of "Cholesterol. And Now the Bad News..." The former features a decidedly unhappy face formed by two over easy eggs and a lovely piece of bacon (who only eats one piece of bacon?!). This faulty science, discussed in the more recent Time piece, made a lot of people in the food industry rich and countless others sick or worse... But the truth of the matter is, your body does indeed need fat, it just needs the right amount. Enter Flexible Eating, which will teach you what is the optimal quantity for you.

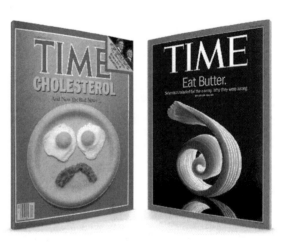

[Figure 7.1]

LET'S LOOK AT SOME OF THE BENEFITS OF FAT:

- **Source of Energy:** Fat provides a secondary source of energy, aside from carbohydrates. When you exercise, you will use carbohydrates for the first twenty minutes of continuous activity. After that, you will tap into fat as a fuel source for activities that will last thirty minutes or more like biking, running and swimming.
- **Vitamins:** Our bodies need micronutrients (vitamins & minerals) as well as macronutrients and fat helps to absorb vitamins that are fat-soluble such as Vitamins A, D, and K.
- **Skin & Hair:** With the help of those fat-soluble vitamins fat helps to keep hair and skin healthy 'n' looking good.
- **Joints:** Because our joints need protection, the essential fatty acids such as omega 3 have been shown to aid in joint health.
- **Weight Loss:** Good news! Fat, much like protein requires a lot of effort from the body to digest and break it down. This extra effort keeps you satiated longer which in turn reduces overconsumption.

Fat, just like protein and carbohydrates, is our *friend* and is a valuable macronutrient. Fat in and of itself will not make you fat. Eating it in *excess*, coupled with a sedentary lifestyle will.

Let's take a moment to focus on that word – **excess**. The aim is to determine how much of each macronutrient your body needs to function optimally based on your activity level and goals. When those macronutrient targets are achieved and paired with exercise, you will no doubt be on the right track toward obtaining the body and performance level you desire.

Soon you'll know your personal macronutrient numbers like the back of your hand. As we go along, I am going to continue teaching you how to use them on a daily basis to achieve your goals and lifestyle in a long-term sustainable way.

Take a break from reading and give yourself a moment or two to digest what you just read. Use this time to think about your eating habits and current relationship with food.

6 What are some hardships you envision yourself encountering as you try to improve your relationship with food?

_____

_____

_____

_____

_____

_____

_____

7 How can you overcome those potential challenges?

_____

_____

_____

_____

_____

_____

_____

_____

CHAPTER 8

GINGER IS IN CONTROL

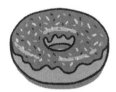

Prior to adopting Flexible Eating, I was definitely a binge eater. Honestly, at times I would just eat because I loved food and not because I was hungry. It all tasted so good and everything I did was purely for pleasure. I ate whatever I wanted, whenever I wanted it, with no recognition of how it would affect my health. It's scary to think about now how that was 41 lbs. ago – things have totally changed!

My goal was simple: to be the best version of myself that I could be every day. That was my mindset for quite a long time, but all I ever did about it was workout; I thought that was enough. I was certainly wrong and experienced an awakening over Memorial Day weekend 2015. My CrossFit gym had just finished the Hero WOD "Murph" and I was devastated to discover I could barely run a mile. Something needed to change and as luck would have it one of my friends mentioned after the workout how she was planning on giving Flexible Eating a shot in an effort to get her nutrition in check.

I thought that a dietary renovation sounded like an amazing idea and figured we would both find success if we stuck to the plan together. Initially, I used her numbers and lost 5 lbs. in a week! That weight loss was great, but the biggest surprise was that I was so full of energy. In the past, whenever I tried to lose weight, it was normally accompanied with feeling sluggish, lethargic, or even bloated – probably because I was not eating enough. I was sold and totally hooked on Flexible Eating; the next week I contacted Jason to obtain my own personalized numbers.

There was definitely a learning curve to overcome in the beginning. I had changed from eating whatever, whenever to being very diligent about hitting my numbers. It took about a month of planning my days ahead of time before I really developed a good rhythm. Luckily, throughout the whole process, I have been immensely fortunate to have the support of my husband. He and I are very social people and our big events usually involve going out to eat on the weekends with friends. The challenge of hitting my numbers was made easier because he would ask me in advance what restaurant I wanted to go to and research the menus online so I could plan ahead.

Before Flexible Eating, I would have said "no way!" to broccoli and opted for quick and easy foods such as smoothies and salads instead. I thought that I was being healthy, but reflecting back on it all now, I realize just one of those salads probably contained my entire days' worth of fat! Now, my taste buds have changed, broccoli is a new friend, and I am making sensible choices in my food selection based off of my numbers.

To speak even further on that, as a business owner, work can be very stressful; and that aspect of my life was negatively affecting my relationship with food. Through this whole process, I have started to look deeper into the **WHY** behind my past eating habits and that knowledge has helped me move past them and into a more fruitful mindset. Now when co- workers bring in brownies or other snacks I have the will power to not eat them or the control to alter my plan for the day and fit a tasty treat into my macros.

Personally, I think that if I had not made the effort to plan out each day ahead of time I would have failed. If there is one piece of advice I can pass along to others – it would be to take that time at the end of every night and plan your meals out for tomorrow. It's a simple, easy thing to do, that just takes ten minutes of your time – it makes all the difference in the world.

Planning helps give me some peace of mind and to not feel guilty about having a handful of gummy bears, instead I can just go into MyFitnessPal and adjust another meal, and the day has not been sabotaged by those sweet 'n' colorful little bears.

I am **EXCITED** about food now. I get pumped up to eat strawberries over cookies because I have exposed myself to a greater variety of foods. I love it; I love having control over this part of my life – and it has been a game changer! I feel empowered and excited about my health and fitness. Flexible Eating has changed my life and I truly believe that if others commit to it, it will change their lives too.

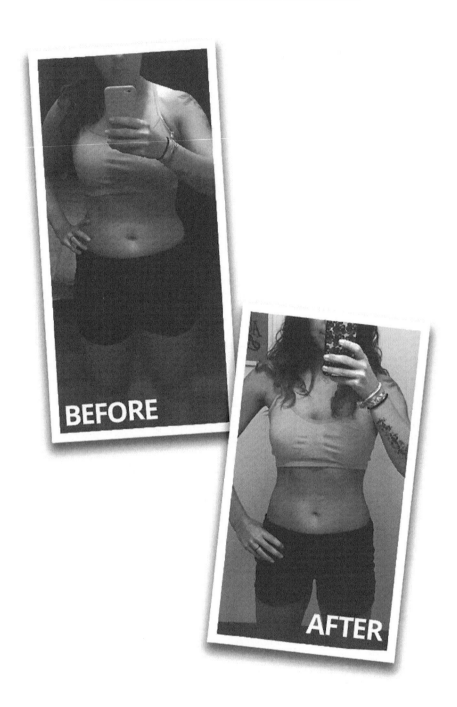

CHAPTER 9

HIT YOUR NUMBERS

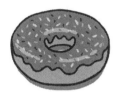

Through eating flexibly, I have finally found enormous success in my own personal fitness journey – but as you may know, it hasn't always been a cake walk. Prior to establishing my own macronutrient numbers, I weighed 170 lbs. and consumed 1,900 calories per day. I felt as though I was on top of my game physically – but that was so not the case. After a year of Flexible Eating my weight was down to 140 lbs. and I currently consume 3,000 calories per day. I look and feel better than ever and I continue to set personal records in my daily fitness. I sleep better and genuinely feel stronger overall.

How can it be that I can eat 1,100 more calories per day and yet be 30 lbs. lighter with better performance and aesthetics? I touched on this briefly in *Chapter 4 – A Word On Metabolism*. I fixed my metabolism by consistently eating the appropriate amount of food for my activity level and goals. I hope you noticed the "c" word there – **CONSISTENTLY!**

And you can do this too – you just need to take the first steps into putting Flexible Eating into practice by finding out your own personalized "numbers."

FLEXIBLE PREGNANCY

As a side note, if you happen to be pregnant – you need to **consult with your doctor before trying Flexible Eating**. Assuming you've done that, there are some important things to consider. Our goal during this time is not weight loss, but is instead a healthy weight gain. Putting on serious amounts of excess weight while pregnant is easy, but we want to limit it to 25 to 35 lbs.

During your pregnancy we would only need to increase a total of 300 calories from what you would normally eat to maintain pre-pregnancy weight. After your bouncing bundle of joy is born, we would want to increase another 200 calories during nursing.

Counting your macros is entirely possible while pregnant – you just have to listen to your body when it's asking for something which is seemingly out of the norm – like a steak smothered in chocolate syrup. The beauty of Flexible Eating is that you can make the changes on the fly as you need to.

Everyone is different when it comes to eating while pregnant. Your hormones are going crazy and when the baby comes it continues to share your body's stored nutrients – so expect to be hungry after nursing! The healthier you are, the healthier your baby will be. Getting pregnant is not an excuse to all of a sudden eat whatever you want. You still need to be sensible about things to ensure you put on that healthy amount of weight.

ACTIVITY LEVEL

Activity Level	Description
Outlier	**You have a medical condition that requires you to eat less calories than the average person as prescribed by your doctor.**
(11)	**Moderate Activity:** Exercises regularly for one hour three to four times per week and works a sedentary job.
12	**Active Exerciser:** Someone who does CrossFit, Weight trains regularly, leads an active lifestyle.
13	**Active Athlete:** Someone who does CrossFit, weight trains, is very active and also plays a sport a few days a week in addition to working out.
14	**Focused Athlete:** Someone who consistently exercises two or more times per day and plays a sport.
15	**Elite Athlete:** Someone whose job it is to exercise, professional CrossFit athlete, endurance athlete, weightlifter.
Outlier	**Olympic Level Athlete, pregnant person, or hard gainer.**

Table 9.1

I really want to emphasize that while CrossFit is mentioned quite a bit in **Table 9.1** – this is **NOT** a "CrossFit diet." I am including CrossFit as a reference point because I realize that a large number of you are coming from a CrossFit background, and using it as a baseline indicator will hopefully help you decide your level of activity more easily. Flexible Eating is a lifestyle for all humans, not just CrossFitters.

When you select your activity level, be as honest as you possibly can be. The vast majority of people I meet with individually, usually end up at either an 11 or 12 activity level. More than likely, that is the range you will fall into.

Go no lower than an 11 activity level as 10 or below would be appropriate for someone who has a medical condition that requires them to eat a much lower amount of macronutrients than the average person – this is a doctor's order only type of situation. The same goes for an activity level of 16 or more. That level of macronutrients is appropriate for olympic level athletes, potentially a pregnant person, or someone who has an extremely difficult time gaining body weight, otherwise known as: "the hard gainer."

FLEXIBLE EATING MACRONUTRIENT EQUATION

After you have ascertained your activity level, it's time to use the Flexible Eating Macronutrient Equation below to calculate your own macronutrient numbers.

STEP 1	STEP 2	STEP 3
Daily Calorie Requirement (DCR)	**Daily Protein Requirement (P)**	**Daily Carbohydrate Requirement (C)**
Goal Weight multiplied by Activity Level	Goal Weight multiplied by 90% for Men or 80% for Women	**(DCR)** multiplied by 10%
= DCR	**= (P) in Grams**	**= (C) in Grams**
Answer: 1980	Answer: 144 132	Answer: 198 198

STEP 4	STEP 5	STEP 6
Daily Fat Requirement (F) Part 1:	**Daily Fat Requirement (F) Part 2:**	**Daily Fat Requirement (F) Part 3:**
(P) in grams plus **(C)** in grams, then multiplied by 4	**(DCR)** minus combined **(P)** and **(C)** calories	**(F)** Fat calories divided by 9
= combined calories from these two macronutrients	**= (F) Fat calories**	**= (F) in Grams**
Answer: 342 1368	Answer: 2322 612	Answer: 258 68

Summary: *(Log your calculated numbers below as you find them).*

Daily Calorie Requirement **(DCR):** 1980

Daily Protein Requirement in Grams **(P):** 144 g

Daily Carbohydrate Requirement in Grams **(C):** 198g

Daily Fat Requirement in Grams **(F):** 68 g

576
712

While there are dozens of formulas out there that you could use to calculate your daily macronutrient numbers, through experience, I have found that mine helps my clients achieve the best possible results. What will ultimately be more important than the formula, is that you are starting at a place that is sensible for you. In other words, you are introducing an awareness to your eating that might not have existed before.

Now that we have outlined the **Flexible Eating Macronutrient Equation** we can break it down into more digestible (*pun definitely intended!*) pieces. Let's use a fictional person by the name of Johanna. She is 32 years old, currently weighs 143 lbs., and is 5'4" tall". She wants to lose weight around her midsection and thighs so that she can fit into clothing she has not been able to wear since college. Johanna goes to the gym four times a week, has a fairly sedentary job working in an office and otherwise does not engage in any regular physical activity.

Johanna's goal weight is **123 lbs**. Based on what we know about her lifestyle, her activity level puts her at an **11**. *(remember **MOST** of you reading this book will either be an **11** or **12** activity level)*. To find Johanna's daily caloric requirement we would multiply **123 lbs.** by an **11** activity level which equals **1,353** calories. If our aim is to eat in a way that supports lean body mass and not excess fat – this is all the daily nutrition Johanna requires to support her goal weight.

I realize some of you might look at that number of calories and think "that doesn't seem like enough food." Well, lets talk big picture here – a great deal of people chronicly undergo a cycle of under eating then over eating. Those dietary habits wreak havoc on the metabolism and actually cause the body to become more prone to storing excess body fat. Our model Johanna – although fictional – is exactly like most people out there. She has poor eating habits which results in her not having the body she wants. Once Johanna starts *consistently* hitting her numbers, her body is going to respond to that change. Committing to Flexible Eating, she will be well on her way to correcting her wayward metabolism.

Now that we've calculated her overall calories, let's focus on the breakdown of her macros. Following the equation, her daily allotment of protein will be **98g** a day (found by multiplying her goal weight of **123 lbs.** by **80%** – please note that daily protein calculation is different for men and women. Refer back to page 65 to be sure that you are using the correct version of the formula when calculating your personal numbers). For many of you, especially women, this will be a much higher amount of protein consumption than you are used to. But hopefully, after reading *Chapter 7 – Building Blocks*, you understand why protein is so important, and why this number is so high!

Next, to find Johanna's carbohydrate needs we multiply her daily calories by **10%**. For Johanna, this means that **1,353** times by **10%** equals **135g** of carbs per day. This might seem like a lot, but remember as you learned previously – carbs are not evil (and they're also usually super delicious).

Finally, to calculate the daily fat intake, we use the data that we have found for protein and carbs. First, Johanna must figure out how many calories she is consuming from those other two macronutrients combined by using the knowledge gained in *Chapter 6 – Flexible Eating, Defined*, that one gram of protein or carbohydrate is equal to 4 calories. So, to calculate how many calories she is getting from protein, we multiply **98g** by 4 and it equals 392 – the number of protein-provided calories. Next up is carbs, where we do the same thing: **135g** times **4** equals **540** calories of carbohydrates. Then we add those two caloric amounts – **392** calories plus **540** which equals **932** calories. Then we want to find out how many calories are designated for fat macros – so we subtract **932** from the total daily calories of **1,353**. This number,

421 is then divided by the number of calories in **one** gram of fat (9) to determine the number of grams of fat needed, which is **47g**. And there you have it!

When you calculate your macros, if you come up with a number such as 110.7, you would round up to 111g. Anything .5 and above is rounded to the nearest number, while anything below .5 is reduced. So, for example 110.3 would be recorded as just 110g.

Here's a pretty diagram of her macros, for all the visual people I lost on that mathematical excursion.

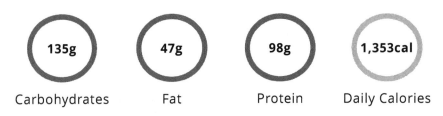

135g	47g	98g	1,353cal
Carbohydrates	Fat	Protein	Daily Calories

Congratulations on getting through the calculations! Take a break from reading and give yourself a moment or two to digest what you just read. Use this time to think about your eating habits and current relationship with food.

8   If you were going to try, I mean **REALLY TRY** to sabotage your own diet, what are three things you would do? Be as detailed as possible with your master plan!

(1) ....

....

....

....

....

....

....

....

(2) ....

....

....

....

....

....

....

....

(3)

_____

_____

_____

_____

_____

_____

_____

_____

(4)

_____

_____

_____

_____

_____

_____

_____

_____

CHAPTER 10

QUALITY

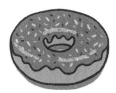

Flexible Eating is **NOT** restrictive in regards to the food that you can eat. There is no food that I will tell you to eliminate or that won't "fit in" with this system. So, if you enjoy eating donuts, then by all means have one. I also don't want to see you emptying out your refrigerator because someone somewhere told you that certain foods were "bad." There are no "bad" foods, there are of course better options, but ultimately it's just the amount of food that you eat that can either be detrimental or beneficial to your health.

When it comes to changing the way you eat, no one likes to go "cold turkey". Trying to instantaneously eliminate the foods that make you happy is an unrealistic expectation. Let's be real, you will eventually have a donut (and probably five more that you won't admit to). It doesn't matter what you call it – a meltdown, a set-back, a cheat day / weekend – it's going to happen. Not only is restricting what you are allowed to eat harmful, but the associated guilt will be damaging to your relationship with food and causes you to essentially demonize it! For these reasons, it would be better to have a donut every day if that is what it takes to keep your nutrition in check 365 days per year.

However, just to be clear, I'm not trying to change conventional science here; you'll never convince me that a donut is a healthier option than broccoli. At the same time though, you need to keep your sanity! And, for a lot of people, this includes having foods that nurture their minds and not just their abs. Establishing a better relationship with food, where you can have one donut without binging, is as crucial a part of Flexible Eating as is meeting your daily numbers.

Plan to eat the things that will make you happy then *eat them*! Flexible Eating allows you to enjoy the foods you love and alleviates the familiar feelings of deprivation, guilt or shame usually associated with these "bad" foods. At the end of the day, you will sleep better knowing you had that donut, and in the morning you will wake up lighter.

With that being said, I'm not giving you an excuse to eat like an asshole. You are *(most likely)* an adult and you know better than to eat fast food or junk for every single meal. The idea is to be flexible, but that shouldn't preclude you from making some **SENSIBLE** decisions. No one wants to get scurvy after all! To avoid disease and vitamin deficiencies, you will still need to make an effort to include foods that are high in micronutrients, while allowing yourself the freedom to enjoy some comfort foods alongside them too. Not only will foods like fruits and vegetables help protect you against disease, but they will also keep you satiated (fuller) longer than most pleasurable foods, because they are so nutrient dense.

FOOD VOLUME

Let's take a closer look at that broccoli vs. a donut scenario; on the left in **Figure 10.1**, we have a plate of Broccoli and to the right a plate of donuts. Both would contribute towards your daily allotment of carbohydrates, but it's the broccoli that will go the extra mile. One bag of Birds Eye steamable broccoli contains: 30 calories, 0g of fat, 20g of carbohydrates, 4g of protein – not to mention all of the vitamins, minerals and fiber. One Dunkin Donuts Boston Kreme Donut comes with: 310 calories, 16g of fat, 39g of carbohydrates, 3g of protein.

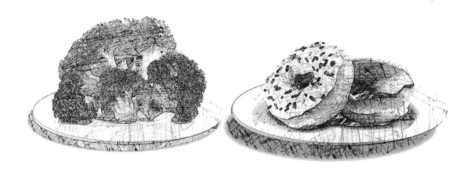

[Figure 10.1]

If we think back to Johanna, who needs to eat 135g of carbohydrates per day, she would need to eat roughly 6 ½ bags of steamable broccoli to fulfill her needs for that macronutrient. On the other hand, she could also meet that requirement by eating 3 ½ donuts – and we all know, no one just eats half a donut! Both scenarios play out with Johanna hitting her daily budget for carbohydrates, but neither is truly ideal – we need to find a balance.

Even though Johanna is achieving her macronutrient goal, the chances are eating only donuts would leave her feeling hungry throughout the day. You may also experience a similar situation and wonder *"why am I so hungry if I am eating more food than I normally do?"* Well, that is because we need to take into consideration **food volume**.

While 6 ½ bags of broccoli and 3 ½ Boston Kremes equal the same amount of carbohydrates, the broccoli is an overall greater amount of food when we pile it all together next to the donuts. Your body would need to put in a considerable amount of work to digest all that broccoli (expending more energy, leading to a higher-level of weight loss) and it will keep you satiated for a longer period of time. Donuts are quick and easy *(I've already eaten three while you read this paragraph!)* and don't make your body work very hard via digestion which results in those hunger pangs coming back sooner than you would desire.

So, broccoli does indeed have its benefits. Nutrient-dense foods like it, should absolutely be incorporated into your diet, but that doesn't necessarily mean that there is no room for donuts as well, what we need is variety. Variety with your food choices is going to be the key to finding that balance in meeting all of your macronutrient requirements. Eating ungodly amounts of broccoli is not realistic and eating only 3 ½ donuts is the easy way out that could in turn make your days more difficult to get through. Instead, have one donut (or whatever treat you wish) at the end of the day while you watch your favorite show; fill the rest of the meals with foods such as apples, baby carrots, breads, melons, oatmeal, pasta, rice, spinach, sweet potatoes and of course broccoli if that's your thing.

Everyone's personal daily menu is going to look a little different, but the goal is to be both sensible and not restrictive. Having the foods you love will help give you peace of mind while mixing in those garden fresh foods will help you feel full and cover all of your bases by giving your body all of the micronutrients such as fiber it needs to achieve your goals. Speaking of fiber...

FIBER

Before we go any further, there's one more nutritional factor that I do like to touch upon which is getting enough fiber. Because I care about you and this so much, I'll share a little personal story to help stress why fiber is so important. When I started eating flexibly, I would log in some of my favorite go-to snacks: Cannoli's, Pop Tarts, Swedish Fish, Twizzlers – all the important stuff. I would hit my numbers **e x a c t l y**. I felt great and was killing workouts. After a few weeks though, I began to realize that I had lost my *"regularity"* and that's not normal. The reason for the sudden stall in my system? I hadn't factored in eating enough fiber-rich foods to support regular bowel movements. A little tweaking to the plan – adding more fruits and veggies helped the problem *"pass."*

My recommendation is 10g of fiber per every 1,000 calories.

SO WHAT IS FIBER AND WHERE DO I GET IT?

Dietary fiber is going to come from fruits, vegetables, whole grains and legumes (things like beans and peanuts). Fiber is the part of the plant or grain that your body cannot digest or absorb so it instead passes through your digestive system virtually intact, and helps to add some "bulk" to your movements. Very important – *trust me.*

Insoluble fiber is what helps to push material through your digestive system and bulks up your stool. If constipation is something you suffer from – having more insoluble fiber can certainly help. Foods that contain this fiber type are: wheat bran, nuts, potatoes, cauliflower, and green beans.

EVEN MORE BENEFITS FROM OUR FRIEND FIBER:

- **Bowel Health:** A healthy bowel is extremely important. No one wants hemorrhoid issues and the proper amount of fiber can help to prevent that by helping your digestive system flow and function properly.

- **Maintain Healthy Body Weight:** Foods that contain a good amount of fiber tend to also be more filling – which could reduce the chance of over eating. You will feel "fuller" for longer periods of time as well.

Take a break from reading and give yourself a moment or two to digest what you just read. Use this time to think about your eating habits and current relationship with food.

9   Thinking deeper on the last question, are you currently sabotaging your own diet?

_____

10   If you are, can you come up with any concrete steps that you think might help yourself?

CHAPTER 11

KRISTY THE VEGETARIAN FISH FIGHTER

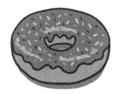

When I was thirteen years old I made the decision to become a vegetarian. This was not only for nutritional reasons, but mainly because I hated the way the animals were being treated. My diet consisted of eating tons of carbs, but very little protein – often a sports bar was it for the day. While I didn't have the guidance I probably needed to pursue vegetarianism correctly; I certainly had the support from my mother, who converted herself so I wouldn't have to go it alone.

In high school I was definitely way too skinny. I would go the entire day without eating any food and then have just one large meal for dinner. My mother would cook a vegetarian dish for the both of us – and another for the rest of the family. None of us knew anything about how much food we really should have been eating and as a result my lifestyle consisted of a cycle of chronic undereating.

Things took a turn for the worse when I went off to college. While I'm sure there was a small celebration in the house at the thought of all the animal products that could be eaten in peace with me gone – I was experiencing a tougher transition myself. At the time, I weighed 120 lbs. at 5'8" and ended up adding meat back into my diet to avoid becoming anemic. On top of that, I tried to navigate university life and all of the typical college diet junk that comes with it on campus.

Eventually, I became increasingly frustrated whenever I stepped on the scale which led me into trying out all sorts of diets including Atkins. So there I was, a former vegetarian – simply lost – following a diet that had me eating tons of meat! On top of that, in order to see the numbers on the scale I wanted, I would workout intensely and dehydrate myself by not drinking water. The whole situation of lacking the knowledge on how to manage my nutrition properly certainly negatively affected my relationship with food.

Things didn't improve after I graduated college and I would continue to chronically under eat. Thinking it would help me make better choices with food, I ended up reverting back to vegetarianism, but all that did was lead me back to a binge carb coma cycle. I weighed 135 lbs., but it was not where I personally wanted to be in terms of my body weight. When that vacation time of the year started to approach, I would limit my calories and start working out to look a little better; when I returned home, everything went back to normal – old habits were always there waiting.

I decided to give Flexible Eating a shot after I saw a friend's success story on Jason's Facebook page. The thought of tracking my macros was intriguing and I hoped it would give me the structure I had been craving. Initially, Flexible Eating was frustrating for me as I have a tendency to be a perfectionist. Not hitting my macros spot on each day definitely bothered me in the beginning to the point where I would hoard the majority of my macros until the end of the day where I could really focus on finishing them. A typical day of eating involved 500 calories between breakfast and lunch and the rest at dinner with my husband. This habit slowly disappeared with practice and eventually finding a nice balance with maintaining my nutrition.

It's funny to think about now – but I was so focused on what I was eating and didn't give a thought to what I wasn't. I had no idea how deficient I was in protein and how wonderfully my body would react when I finally gave it the correct amount. When I first started Flexible Eating, I was 146 lbs. and I currently weigh 120 lbs. My starting calories were 1,200 at the beginning and now I am over 2,000. I've never eaten this much food in my life!

Now, since I'm such a creature of habit, I plan my days ahead of time and try to get in at least half of my days' worth of protein at breakfast. In the beginning all I would think about was "how am I going to eat this much food?" Now at 2,000 calories a day; I have no problem eating every last delicious morsel. My body tells me now when it's hungry and I abide.

My biggest breakthrough has definitely been my mindset. I became a true believer within the first week when I saw the changes in my body all while eating foods I wanted to eat like Oreos and ice cream – **AND** without all the guilt. Another big plus is that when I started I was a size 6 or 8 in most things, but now I'm a size 0. My old clothes fit so loosely I look like a kid wearing her mom's hand-me-downs.

If you're new to Flexible Eating, my advice is to cut yourself some slack. I was really hard on myself at first, but you don't need to be. Give it time. Not every day is going to be perfect, but you can always get back on track the next. All great things worth having will take time.

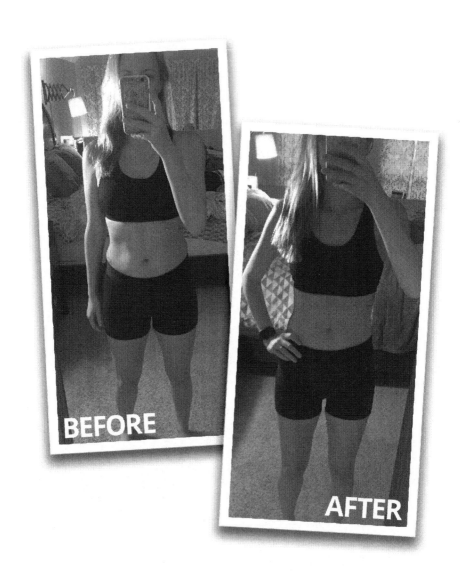

CHAPTER 12

TIMING

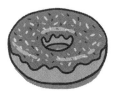

As a flexible eater, the main components you need to focus on are:

- Making a habit of planning ahead and tracking (guidance coming in *Chapter 15 - MyFitnessPal*).
- Consistently consuming the correct number of macros (no days of chronic under or overeating).

As you draw closer to your goals or when you hit a plateau (we'll get to this later) **THEN** you can start to look deeper into the finer details such as nutrient timing, supplementation, and maybe even a little more tweaking of what types of foods you're eating to dial in your results.

But make no mistake, consistently hitting the numbers takes precedence over all this other stuff.

Though meal timing is one of the last things you need to worry about, it is still worth it to discuss in some detail. So, let's talk about some different methods.

PRE-WORKOUT MEALS

A pre-workout meal is meant to be consumed two to three hours before a training session. The goal is to provide more energy for the workout by adding to, or replenishing, your body's glycogen stores. Ideally, you would eat a moderate amount of protein and carbohydrates that are lower on the glycemic index *(a rating system that classifies foods on a scale of 1 to 100 based on how they affect blood-sugar-levels)* so that they will slowly release into the bloodstream and provide energy later on during your activity.

- **Low Level GI Foods (55 and below):** apples, beans, corn tortilla, green leafy vegetables, mangos, peaches, quinoa.
- **Medium Level GI Foods (56 to 69):** banana, cream of wheat, grapes, Kraft Mac & Cheese, raisins.
- **High Level GI Foods (70 and above):** breakfast cereals, fruit roll-up, pretzels, watermelon, white potatoes.

Protein from sources such as egg whites or low fat yogurt, which are easily digestible are excellent. Try to avoid having protein sources like steak (which is high in fat as well) before your workout because it requires more time and effort on the part of the body to break it down. I would suggest keeping fat intake of any kind as low as possible shortly before a workout, as it takes the longest to digest and can also upset your stomach during intense activity.

Example Pre-Workout Meal: Omelet (one serving of egg whites, onions, peppers, a low fat cheese), with some fruit or oatmeal on the side.

POST-WORKOUT MEALS

A post-workout meal should ideally be consumed within 30 to 60 minutes of your training session. No worries, though, if you have to wait longer than that (you will not die or lose #gainz)! After activity your body is craving nutrition, and will readily utilize the nutrients you take in, even if two or three hours have passed.

Ideally this meal would be comprised of protein and carbohydrates. Remember, proteins are the building blocks used to repair the muscles we damage during exercise in order to make them bigger and stronger. The carbohydrates help to guide the protein to the muscles by prompting an influx of insulin into the bloodstream.

Insulin is a "storage hormone" often thought of negatively because of the role it plays in gaining excess fat that we discussed in *Chapter 7 – Building Blocks*. But, insulin does much more than that, and even works in direct opposition to this in some cases! After intense exercise, our bodies are in an extremely insulin-sensitive state. Carbohydrates in a post-workout meal will prompt the release of insulin which will act as the key to unlocking storage centers in the muscles. This is how we will replenish glycogen stores, and shuttle amino acids (protein) to muscles to recover from a workout and grow stronger.

Example Post-Workout Meal: Grilled Chicken accompanied by sweet (or even white!) potato, with some vegetables on the side.

INTERMITTENT FASTING

Intermittent Fasting involves eating all of your daily macronutrients within a specific, often short, timeframe. One example would be fasting for 16 hours and then eating all of your meals within an 8-hour window. This can be done out of convenience, especially if you have a job with limited structured breaks. This method can also be used as a way of sort of shocking your metabolism in the case of plateauing.

Basically, what I want you to get from this is that there is no one singular way to organize your meals. Try not to get ahead of yourself in the beginning, and don't get too caught up in trying to add this scheduling component into what will already likely be a large change to your way of eating. You're not locked into a my-way or the high-way program to organize your meals around your life. At the start, it's not going to be perfect, but if you focus on hitting the numbers and being consistent, it will get better with practice. There's no need to over-think the process until you have a legitimate need for a change.

Take a break from reading and give yourself a moment or two to digest what you just read. Use this time to think about your eating habits and current relationship with food.

11   When do you normally eat your meals? List all the typical times and places. Discuss what your meals actually look like in terms of quantity – it might shock you how little food you actually eat throughout the day.

TIME	PLACE	QUANTITY

TIME	PLACE	QUANTITY

CHAPTER 13

SUPPLEMENTS

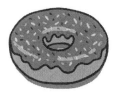

Hitting your numbers with "whole" (i.e. unprocessed) foods can be a difficult task, but it should definitely be your priority in the beginning of your Flexible Eating journey. Yes, you can still achieve results by using protein powder to reach your daily protein requirements for that macronutrient, but at what cost? You would lose out on all of the benefits that real protein sources such as beef, chicken, or fish give you! Powder can't give you the same results of feeling fuller longer, experiencing the thermogenic (fat burning!) process of breaking down those nutrients, and the abundance of added vitamins and minerals the non-manufactured sources provide. Our society is wrapped up in "quick 'n' easy" fixes – but nutrition shouldn't be one of them. We should give it as much care, deliberation, and thought that we can!

However, there are always exceptions to the rule. If you have had success eating more whole foods than you were previously, but are still falling short of hitting your daily macronutrient requirements, then supplementing may have to be an option. But keep in mind, these are called "supplements" for a reason; they should not comprise the bulk of your daily menu by any means.

PROTEIN POWDER

Protein powder is the most popular supplement on the planet. Almost everyone, at some point, finds a need for it – whether it be to lose weight, gain weight, or just to flavor a smoothie. To complement this high demand, there is an equally huge supply; there are many different types of protein powder such as:

- **General Whey:** Your everyday whey protein is meant to be used for snacks or for beefing up meals. You can use it to hit your numbers at the end of the day if you just cannot bare to eat one more morsel of turkey breast or Greek yogurt – but just be sure to do your best to not rely on it *too* much.
- **Post-Workout:** This type of protein powder is made from whey protein isolates that are fast absorbing – which is definitely what you want post workout. Be sure to check the labels and read up on what kind of protein powder you are buying. Some, such as Casein, are slow digesting and designed to be taken at night before you go to bed to give the body a consistent stream of amino acids while you sleep. So, it would not be ideal post-workout.
- **Weight Gainer:** These protein powder products *(try saying that five times fast!)* are jam packed with macronutrients – often being upwards of 500 to 600 calories per shake! This is not something I recommend a flexible eater should rely on. You take in a bulk of calories in one shot, and you will miss out on all the important

digestive processes that happen when you eat whole foods. Also, we again need to think about food volume, the minimal volume associated with weight gainer protein will not help in keeping you satiated for very long.

For flexible eaters, I would recommend protein powder to be used mainly to replenish the body post workout. Ideally, no more than one serving per day and it should only use up roughly 21g of your daily protein.

FISH OIL

Sounds kind of gross, doesn't it?

Trust me, it's really not that bad. In fact, fish oil is an outstanding supplement that you should especially be taking if you are involved in rigorous exercise. Fish oil is a type of fatty acid that comes from the body tissue of oily fish such as anchovies, salmon, and tuna. White meat fish such as cod, haddock, and pollock also contain these fatty acids, but in much smaller amounts. When you eat these fish they supply your body with essential omega-3 fatty acids. The big two are:

- Eicosapentaenoic acid (EPA)
- Docosahexaenoic acid (DHA)

Tongue-twisters, to say the least!

If you consume a pretty high amount of fatty, oily fish like salmon, then you are probably good to go. On the other hand, if you are someone who shies away from the slippery little fellas, you might want to consider picking up a bottle of fish oil!

SOME BENEFITS FROM FISH OIL:

- **Healthy Cholesterol:** Fish oil helps to support healthy blood cholesterol levels that are already within a normal rage.
- **Stronger Bones:** As we age, strengthening our bones becomes more and more important. Fish oil has been shown to greatly aid in this (especially in women who are entering their menopausal years). At that time women are no longer naturally producing the levels of hormones (such as estrogen) they used to, their bones can thin and lose strength with time. Because of that, they are at a greater risk for illnesses such as osteoporosis. Fish oil can help to increase bone density, and offset calcium imbalances!

Needless to say fish oil is pretty important. Take a good hard look at how you feel, what you are eating, and your aching bones. Chances are fish oil can help. It's also a major bang for your supplement buck in that it will take care of a lot of issues at the same time.

VITAMIN B6

It's time to get sciencey again! Vitamin B6 is a very important micronutrient that is necessary to help regulate levels of a compound called homocysteine in your body.

Homocysteine is an amino acid that is found within your blood. A high level of this protein in the bloodstream has been linked to the development of heart and blood vessel disease...those things that can cause heart attacks.

If you do not take in enough of our friend B6, the large quantities of homocysteine in blood can cause inflammation and damage blood vessel linings. Then, before you know it, plaque builds up in your arteries which can definitely lead to a heart attack or a stroke. *Not good.*

That right there alone is a pretty stellar reason to supplement with Vitamin B6, but the other benefits are great too:

- **Healthy Brain Function:** Vitamin B6 helps to support proper brain functions. A lack of dietary B6 has been shown to be linked to diseases such as Alzheimer's and Dementia in older populations.
- **Happy Hormones:** Supplementing with Vitamin B6 can help to improve your mood! With it, the body creates those feel good hormones serotonin and norepinephrine. So, if you're down in the dumps all the time, you may just be low on the B6.
- **PMS:** Basically, everyone is familiar (in some way) with what these three nasty little letters stand for: Premenstrual Syndrome. B6 has been found to have a positive effect on neurotransmitters in the brain that are in charge of pain management, you might be experiencing a particularly rough time of the month (either personally or by association) because of low levels of B6.
- **Restful Nights:** Vitamin B6 can help you sleep better by aiding the body in creating melatonin. If you have trouble sleeping, adding this into your diet might be a good place to start!

So, vitamin B6, just like the rest of the micronutrients we are going to talk about, is indeed quite crucial for your health and overall emotional well-being. Handy little pills are convenient, for sure, but you can get it naturally from places such as...

- **Proteins:** Beef, Beef Liver, Chicken Breast, Chickpeas, Lean Pork, Tuna, Turkey Breast, and Pinto Beans.
- **Nuts:** Pistachios, Sesame Seeds, Sunflower Seeds.
- **Fruits & Veggies:** Avocados, Bananas, Prunes, Spinach.

VITAMIN D

For all the desk jockeys, keyboard warriors and vampires out there who spend your days indoors slumped in front of a computer screen – you're probably in need of Vitamin D. If you want to live longer, perform better in 'n' out of the gym and look better naked (let's be real – this is really what it is *all* about), this supplement will be a game changer.

Here's why:

- **Strong Bones:** Vitamin D helps to keep your bones strong and reduces your risk of osteoporosis as you age. You don't want to be frail and brittle in your golden years do you? Of course not! The goal is to live independently with vibrant energy, all your original teeth and a head full of sexy silver hair. After all, everything we do (being active, taking care of our diet, getting enough Vitamin D) is essential to ensure a long, happy, broken-bone free life.
- **Immune System:** No one wants to be stuck on the couch, drugged up on Dayquil, watching Full House reruns while hacking up a lung and littering the floor with used tissues. Enter Vitamin D. This vitamin helps regulate your immune system by reducing the

inflammatory response to infections. Save those sick days for the beach, not the couch!

- **Performance:** Vitamin D is necessary for the absorption of calcium, which plays a huge role in maintaining bone 'n' muscle form and function. Your body uses it to help with the process of muscle contraction and other physiological functions. If you're **a.)** not eating foods that are rich in calcium (i.e. green leafy veggies) and / or **b.)** not getting enough Vitamin D to absorb calcium; then your body might need to go elsewhere to get it for proper muscle function – (leaching from your bones). If you are an athlete who wants to bust their butt in the gym, skipping out on the Vitamin D or veggies could cost you in the long run. In this scenario, your body will steal the calcium it needs to support your high level activity, right from your own bones!

FUN IN THE SUN:

Exposing your bare skin to the sun is the best way to get Vitamin D and the more skin the sun touches the better. Now, this does not mean you should be spending hours upon hours burning or even tanning your skin to get Vitamin D. In as little as 15 minutes your body can produce 10,000 to 25,000 IU (International Units). How fast you actually produce Vitamin D depends on your skin color, the time of day and where you live.

Studies have found that people with pale skin produce Vitamin D much faster than those who are darker – **BUT** that also may mean that you probably burn faster – so be careful! At the same time, lathering on too much sun screen does make it harder for your body to make that precious Vitamin D, because the same rays that you're protecting yourself from are also the ones delivering this important vitamin. Fortunately, it is extremely difficult to "overdose" on D, and your body will naturally stop producing it when it makes enough, so no worries there.

Very few foods contain Vitamin D, which is why contact with the sun or supplementations are going to be your best sources. In a perfect world you would be able to be outside at about mid-day to get your fix, as studies have shown that to be the best time for exposure. But, that's not always realistic when you have a job where you can't get away in the middle of the workday. Living close to the equator helps a lot, too, with that whole year-round- fun-in-the-sun deal. Sorry Seattleites...

OUR OLD FRIEND, FAT:

As I mentioned before, all three of the macronutrients are important, *including* fat. Your body needs Fat in order to absorb Vitamin D. So, if you're shying away from the big F you could be missing out on getting enough D.

VITAMIN C

Vitamin C is another helpful micronutrient for ensuring overall health, and for looking your best in your birthday suit. Foods that are rich in the Big C include, but are not limited to:

- **Veggies:** Broccoli, Bell Peppers, Brussel Sprouts, Cauliflower, Kale, and Mustard Greens (mustard on your hot dog, delicious – yes, but not the same), Onions, Parsley, Spinach
- **Fruits:** Apricots, Cantaloupe, Grapefruit, Kiwi, Lemons, Limes, Mangos, Oranges, Pineapple, Strawberries, Tangerines, Tomato (yep, a fruit), and Watermelon
- **Berries:** Blackberries, Raspberries, and Strawberries

> *Anyone else suddenly in the mood for an
> ice-cold tropical smoothie?*

BENEFITS:

- **Immune System:** Vitamin C is important for flexible eaters to maintain their immune systems. A healthy dose of Vitamin C will help you protect your body from infections and fight against harmful bacteria and viruses. It can also serve as an effective antihistamine that can reduce the symptoms of the common cold – inflammation, stuffy nose and body aches.

- **Antioxidants:** Vitamin C is a powerful antioxidant which protects your body from free radicals that cause oxidative stress or "cellular rust" – that can lead to conditions such as heart disease and strokes – some pretty serious stuff! Free radicals have also been linked to colon, esophagus, lung, mouth, stomach and throat cancer.

- **Protect Your Heart:** Speaking of cardiovascular disease, Vitamin C has been shown to reduce the chances of hypertension. It can also aid in the dilation of blood vessels which in turn will help prevent serious diseases such as atherosclerosis, high cholesterol and congestive heart failure.

- **Other Cool Perks:** The benefits of the Big C are plentiful. It helps maintain healthy bones, teeth and connective tissue within the body. It speeds up the ability to heal from wounds. And let's not overlook the fact that Vitamin C also helps our eyes to function as well! Deficiencies can lead to cataracts (blurry vision) – Big C fights against this by increasing the blood flow to the eyes.

MAGNESIUM

I know, I know it's tough; not everyone likes to eat their fair share of veggies! But that is most likely why you and half of the U.S. population are not getting enough of the powerhouse magnesium. Magnesium is a heavy hitter in the micronutrient world – it's essential for more than 300 enzymatic processes in your body, from breaking down food to pumping blood through your heart.

Magnesium also plays an important role in how your muscles move by monitoring tension and helping to relax your muscle fibers between contractions. In addition to that, this wonderful micronutrient can increase sleep time and quality by promoting high melatonin levels within the body. This allows you to sleep more soundly and reduce stress.

BRONX VANILLA

Fun fact! Waaaay back in the day, the slang term for Garlic was Bronx Vanilla. Now, I know what you're thinking – "Hey, Garlic is not a supplement." Well, while that's *technically* (I guess) correct, I eat a raw clove of Garlic every day just like I take my fish oil. I wholeheartedly believe that it helps keep me and my body operating at 100% and I'll tell ya why...

TOP 10 REASONS I EAT GARLIC EVERYDAY:

1. **Prevents Heart Attacks:** Garlic contains an antioxidant called allicin that aids in preventing heart attacks and strokes. It is only produced when you crush the garlic clove and it instantaneously neutralizes free radicals. That's a pretty darn big deal right there.

2. **Lowers Blood Pressure:** Eating crushed garlic can immediately lower your blood pressure. I have read some studies that reported blood vessels relaxing up to 75% after eating that delicious Bronx Vanilla.

3. **Fight the Common Cold:** I rarely get sick – honestly could not remember the last time I was laid up on my couch stuffy nosed and miserable. The nutrients inside of Garlic have been found to strengthen and aid the immune system to resist illness.

4. **Liver Detox:** Garlic releases toxins from the liver.

5. **Blood Clots:** Nature's baby aspirin helps to thin blood and prevent blood clots.

6. **Hair Loss:** For you gentlemen out there who suffer from premature hair loss – Garlic has been found to stop it! That awesome antioxidant allicin is the hero again and why I have such long luscious locks of hair.

7. **Cold Sores:** It helps to heal cold sores and reduce swelling in the body.

8. **Athletes Foot:** Garlic is a natural antifungal. Soaking your feet in warm water with Garlic just might be the trick you need to get rid of a case of it!

9. **Weight Loss:** Reduce fat stores in the body with your new best friend, Garlic!

10. **Aids against Impotence:** Need I say more??

PUORI

To recap, supplements should be the sidekick not the hero. Do your best to get as many macro- and micronutrients from real foods as possible; we don't want to be getting any more than 20% of our daily protein from powders. Vitamin C is also a must! So do your best to work those green leafy veggies and citrus fruits into your meals alongside those donuts and ice cream.

Aside from that, I highly recommend you cover your bases and supplement with Vitamin D, Magnesium, and Zinc. I personally recommend checking out the Puori-3 daily pack. It is a complete health supplement system containing all those important micronutrients: 2,000mg Omega-3, 300mg Magnesium, 15mg Zinc, 11mg B6, and 2,500IU Vitamin D3.

I want to stress that I only recommend what I *personally use*, and this pack is something I take every night before I go to bed. It helps me take all of the guesswork out of supplementing. The product was designed with athletes in mind to help you better recover from workouts and life.

The three-piece system (minerals, fish oil, vitamins) is designed with the highest quality materials. Their fish oil has the equivalent amount of omega-3s as is found in four servings of fish! If you're not regularly eating fatty fish, this supplement will definitely ensure you are getting enough healthy omegas.

What's more, Puori sources their fish from Friends of the Sea sustainable fisheries off the coast of Chile and the product is regularly tested by third-party organizations to make sure a high five-star standard is maintained. As an added bonus, they combine their Vitamin D with organic virgin coconut oil to help you get the maximum absorption benefits.

The Puori-3 Health Essentials box comes with 30 servings – the perfect monthly dose. Visit www.Puori.com to purchase this awesome product!

Oh, and don't forget to eat your Garlic!

Take a break from reading and give yourself a moment or two to digest what you just read. Use this time to think about your eating habits and current relationship with food.

12   Do you eat out of boredom? (It's a habit countless people have, so don't feel bad). If yes, what are some ways you think you can break this habit?

_____

_____

_____

_____

_____

_____

_____

_____

_____

_____

_____

_____

_____

_____

_____

_____

_____

CHAPTER 14

JOE FROM STRENGTHLETE

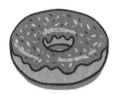

To understand why I started Strengthlete, you need to first know a few details about my life. From 2002 to 2006, I competed in Olympic-style weightlifting at a high-level.

At the peak of my career I took home a bronze medal at the Arnold Classic. In front of a crowd of 3,000 people, I had put together my best meet ever. Six months later, a nagging wrist injury took a turn for the worse and my days on the weightlifting platform were over.

Fast forward to June 2015 and depression had sunk its ugly claws into my life. I weighed 235 lbs., which was a huge deal for me since it's the most I ever weighed in my life. I remember looking down in disbelief at the scale in a hotel room in Denver. "How did this happen?" I thought. I had gained 50 lbs. since leaving college eight years prior.

On top of that, I was in terrible financial shape. I had quit my job to start my own business and genuinely believed I would be a millionaire instantly. Instead, I was working more than ever and racked up $40,000 in credit card debt. How could I be working more hours than ever and not making money? And how did I get this fat? Where did the time go?

When I came back from Colorado, I decided to call my friend and Flexible Eating guru Jason Ackerman. I had seen a ton of before and after pictures posted on his Facebook page and wanted to know more about his methods. In the back of my mind still, I thought I could never be one of those people, but at this point, I saw no other options.

Jason explained to me how Flexible Eating worked and an hour later I got started. I couldn't help but blurt out loud during our phone call "Oh God here we go again – another diet!"

"No, not another diet," Jason emphatically said. "I need to be real with you, Joe. You have to change the way you think about food or you're wasting time." He counselled me for another hour, despite my attempts to get off the phone! He was persistent.

I went from weighing 235 lbs. to 195 lbs. in just under a year. Physically, I lost 40 lbs., but the more important change during that time was what I gained. For the first time in my life, I can buy a bag of peanut M&M's and not have to finish the bag. Even better, I don't want to. I'm not scared of going out to eat with my friends, fearing I won't be able to control myself. I can – for the first time since I was a kid – enjoy eating again.

I started Strengthlete because fitness and nutrition have changed my life. They made me feel capable again, capable enough to make changes that I was scared to do. For the first time in five years, I felt hopeful that the future could be better – more than just scraping by and paying the bills.

Many of you are probably like me – you value health and fitness, but your lives are moving at lightning speed. Work keeps piling higher, the emails never stop rolling in, and you probably feel like there aren't enough hours in the day to do it all.

Taking care of your health just feels like another thing to do. Even though you know it's not the best choice, grabbing lunch or a snack from Starbucks or the nearest vending machine is convenient, and so you do it. This happens because no one is perfect. **But here's the thing, nutrition isn't about being perfect. It's about making better decisions and looking at food without judgement.** That's what Jason taught me.

And you don't need to change everything to succeed. You can start with just one small, good decision followed by another one and then another one right after that. Step by step. This is how we build momentum. It's also how we create lasting change.

Every product we make at Strengthlete is rooted in nutrition. We have built a library of simple and easy to use tools to help you make a better decision, melt away those pounds, increase weight on the barbell, and move faster on those runs. It doesn't matter what your ultimate goal is – whether it's improving your performance as an athlete or simply having more energy to be a better mom, dad, sister, brother, husband or wife. Nutrition goes way beyond the doors of the gym. Your longevity depends on it.

As my gift to you, my fellow flexible eaters, use the discount code **ACKERMAN10** at the checkout when you visit **www.strengthlete.com**.

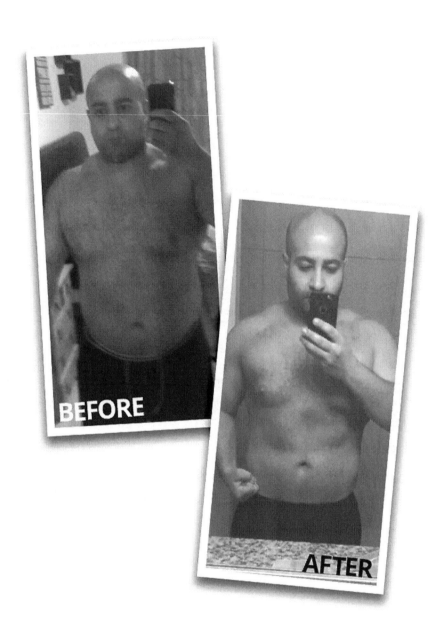

CHAPTER 15

MYFITNESSPAL

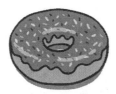

I remember *back in the day*, before cell phones, tablets and apps were common place, all I had was a piece of paper, a pencil and my trusty Texas Instruments calculator. That certainly would have made tracking calories and macronutrients a challenge. Fortunately for you, we have now firmly entered the digital age and are afforded the luxury, convenience, and benefits of new technology such as the popular app MyFitnessPal. Along with your food scale and Tupperware collection, this app will be an important tool towards achieving your short-term and long-term goals.

STEP ONE - GO PREMIUM OR GO HOME

MyFitnessPal is a free app that you can download on both iPhone & Android devices. Once the app is downloaded on your smartphone you will be presented with the option to purchase the "premium" version. If you are serious about pursuing a Flexible Eating lifestyle – I recommend you do it.

Pay now or pay later basically. Invest a little extra now to keep from ultimately spending more in the long run, health-wise. The premium version will give you access to all of its upgraded features. Not to worry, you will without a doubt get your money's worth.

Disclaimer: I am in no way affiliated with this app or any other smartphone fitness tracker. This is just what I personally use as my number one tool and know how important it is in my daily life.

The premium app service offers many additional perks over the free version. The ones that are most important to us are:

- The ability to adjust goal macronutrients by the **gram** instead of just by percentage.
- The useful display of remaining macronutrients on the home screen.

Those two items are essential to planning ahead, tracking your macronutrients throughout the day, and ensuring accuracy in meeting your daily goals, and just general ease of use.

STEP TWO - CUSTOMIZING MYFITNESSPAL

Figure 15.1 depicts the app's default home screen and currently shows you a daily allotment of calories. While that is nice for some people...it's not what we as flexible eaters ultimately want; we need the macros, not the calories. Follow along with me to customize MyFitnessPal to be more suitable for Flexible Eating.

Notice, on **Figure 15.1**, the three dots hovering above the remaining calories that are highlighted in green text – click on them. The link will take you to the change summary screen as seen in **Figure 15.2**, where you can change what is presented on your home screen. Select Macronutrients and the app will auto-save and update by itself.

Your new home screen should now look exactly like the image in **Figure 15.3** (minus the particular numbers of course). These four large circles displaying Carbohydrates, Fat, Protein, and Calories will help you track and hit your numbers each day with ease. As you add meals into the app the numbers within each circle will reduce in correlation to what you input. Whether you have numbers remaining, perfect zeroes, or go over into the negative. It will all be valuable information that you can use to be more successful the next day.

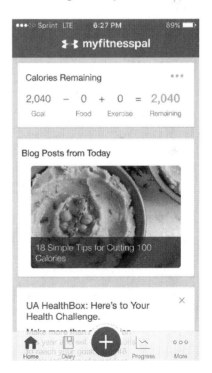

[Figure 15.1]

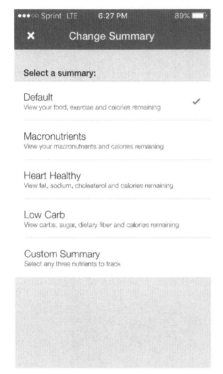

[Figure 15.2]

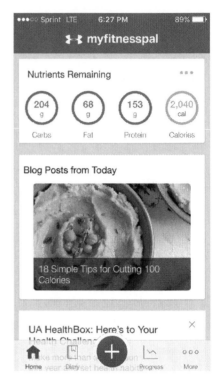

[Figure 15.3]

STEP THREE - UPDATING YOUR NUMBERS

Next, we need to go over how to input your personal macronutrient numbers which were handily calculated in *Chapter 9 – Hit Your Numbers*. If you skipped that step, go back and use the equation to find your daily macronutrient needs based on your goal weight and activity level so that we are all on the same page *(pun intended!)*.

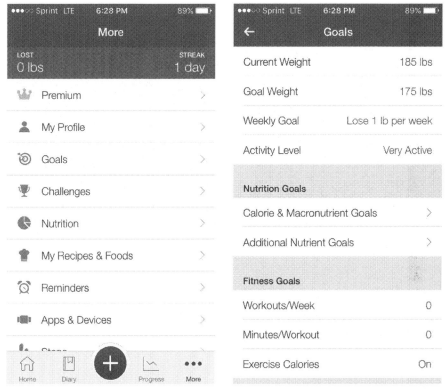

[Figure 15.4]   **[Figure 15.5]**

When you have your numbers ready to go, click on the **"More"** button found on the lower right-hand side of the app's navigation bar. *Now, this information is based on iPhones – which is what I own – but the menu option should be in the upper left hand corner of most Samsung devices in a little drop down menu.* This button will take you to the screen seen in **Figure 15.4**. When you're there click the **"Goals"** button. On the next screen, click **"Calorie & Macronutrient Goals"** as seen in **Figure 15.5**. This is where we will actually be able to update your numbers within the app.

On the Calorie & Macronutrient Goals screen, click either Carbs, Protein, or Fat to bring up the editor. **Figure 15.6** depicts how you can now scroll through a range of numbers to select your desired number of grams. The app will (thankfully) do the math for you and update the calorie count accordingly. Oh! Be sure to **select grams**, as your app may be set to percentage (%) as a default. Then, all you have to do is save your settings, by clicking the little white checkmark, and return to the home screen where you should now see those numbers displayed.

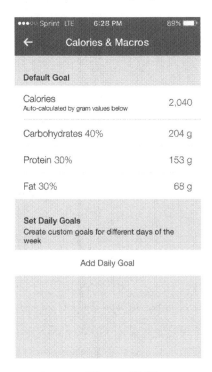

[Figure 15.6]

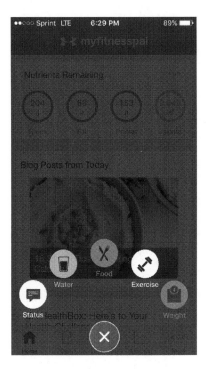

[Figure 15.7]

STEP FOUR - LOGGING FOOD & MEALS

Now the real fun begins! To log and track your food hit the big blue button that can be seen in **Figures 15.1** or **15.3**. It will take you to the screen depicted in **Figure 15.7**. Now that we're here, it is very important to discuss the fact that you should change very little in the basic form of the app. If you use it to track your exercise, weight, or walking steps with something like a FitBit the app will automatically change your daily macronutrient numbers because it will calculate that you need more or less food based on those activities. You definitely do **NOT** want this alteration because we already took your activity level into account when we used the formula to find your numbers. **The app should be used only to track food, nothing else.**

After you select the orange food button – also select the meal you want to input into the app. You will be given options for Breakfast, Lunch, Dinner, or Snacks. For our example we will work on Breakfast.

On the Breakfast screen shown in **Figure 15.8** (and on other subsequent screens) you will have the following options:

- **Select a Recent Meal:** This is a very handy option if you frequently eat meals comprised of the same foods. As long as you keep the portion sizes the same (or remember to alter them) you can easily select the already saved meal again and again each day!
- **Search for Food:** Maybe you preemptively threw away the nutrition label for the chicken breast you recently purchased? No big deal! You can search the app for the exact brand, or for a similar item.
- **Bar Code Scanner:** If you are on the go, or simply appreciate convenience, you can quickly scan a food item's bar code to track and log its nutritional information.
- **Create a New Food:** Add new food items or meals manually.

Our next focus will be that **"Create a New Food"** option. To practice, grab anything in your kitchen that has a nutrition label and let's log it into the app together. Start by clicking the button shown in **Figure 15.8.**

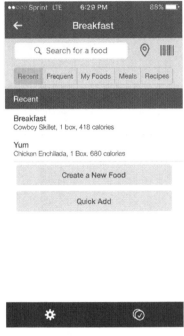

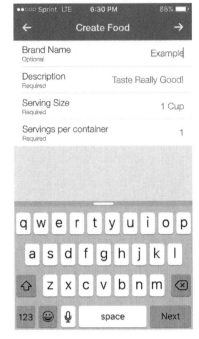

[Figure 15.8]   **[Figure 15.9]**

Next, on the screen shown in **Figure 15.9**, give the food item a brief description. This may be a phrase like "Mama's Fav Casserole" or in the case of a meal it could just be its main ingredients like "chicken, bacon, ranch" *(that sounds pretty good)*. Let your creative juices fly here! After you've input a suitable title, you will need to put in what you will use for the measurement of one serving – this can be in things such as cups, bottles, ounces, or boxes. Finally, you can input how many servings are contained within one container – there may be something like five, 2-cup servings in a pan of Mama's Fav Casserole.

Once this information has been submitted you will be taken to a page where you can input the specific caloric and macronutrient information of the food item. Make sure you record the total calories, carbohydrates, fat and protein for **one** serving then hit the checkmark on the upper right hand-side of the screen to save the information.

Note that adding a food item this way will **automatically** record it for the day and deduct the macronutrients from your daily allotment. Go back to the home screen and check it out!

MyFitnessPal has many options available to make recording data (and thus life) easier and now that we have covered the basics of creating a new food item we can discuss the other tabs shown in **Figure 15.8** that will allow you to input food items into the app. "**My Foods**" is another button that will take you to the "**Create a New Food**" page. "**Meals**" is a section within the app where you can allocate a title to frequent foods that you pair together. For example, on Sundays you typically eat a bagel, two slices of bacon, one egg and 1 ounce of Kraft cheddar cheese. You can save this meal and give it a title such as "Sunday Breakfast Sandwich" so you can use it in the future as a shortcut instead of having to type in each food item separately. "**Recipes**" - is a little easier to use on your computer, but it can also be used on your phone. Here you can import recipes from websites, make adjustments to the ingredients specifying the exact brand and quantities you choose to use and save it with whatever title you like, for example "Food Network's Sweet Potato Waffle.

STEP FIVE - ACTUALLY USE MYFITNESSPAL

So I wasn't joking when I said how powerful a tool MyFitnessPal is, and should be in your new macro-life. Allowing it to do all of the nitty-gritty heavy lifting (storing foods & meals, tracking the daily numbers, and helping you plan ahead) will aid you greatly in achieving your goals. We will go over more specifics on how you can use the app to optimize your day later; but for now just know that using MyFitnessPal is a nutritional game changer that you should take advantage of every day.

Need more guidance on using MyFitnessPal? *Head on over to* **www.ownyoureating.com** – *we frequently post new videos there filled with tips n' tricks on how to use the app.*

Take a break from reading and give yourself a moment or two to digest what you just read. Use this time to think about your eating habits and current relationship with food.

13   Are there any odd places you snack or eat your meals – such as in your car or at your desk at work? Where are these places?

CHAPTER 16

GETTING STARTED

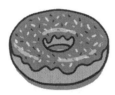

By now you should be excited! Hell, I am so excited for you that I can hardly contain myself! I want to reach right through this page and give you a fist bump! You are taking serious steps towards enacting a new, fruitful lifestyle that will get you the body you have always wanted, while eating the foods you love and all the while keeping your sanity.

But, I want to be real with you. Achieving results from Flexible Eating is definitely going to require hard work on your part. I can give you every tool to help, I can give you a year's worth of planned meals; but I can't pick you up and make you do this. That has to be your choice. As an adult, you've got to take ownership of your decisions. You have a choice every morning when you start a new day; so choose to be a doer – not just a sayer.

Every day, especially in the beginning, you will need to put in concerted effort toward hitting your daily macronutrient requirements and I'll be honest with you – not every day is going to be perfect. My own journey is certainly not easy and I have (and will have) slips just like you will. Welcome to being a human-freaking-being – give yourself a little leeway in the process! Learn to accept the facts that you need to put in the hard work, that achieving your goals will **TAKE TIME** (no quick-fixes here), and that – *to stay on the cliché train* – you will probably appreciate your results that much more when you actually worked hard for them.

Aside from putting in some hard work, you're going to need to trust the process and trust that I've got your back. Because I care about you and want to see you succeed, I'm going to make your life easier for you by giving you this very simple, step-by-step method to getting your flexible eating journey started.

USE THE APP

I know I just talked about this, but using the app is extremely important. Make the investment and let this invaluable tool help you every day. We both know that you more than likely already spend a good deal of time on your phone. Some of it can definitely be dedicated towards managing your nutrition.

PLANNING AHEAD

By failing to prepare, you are preparing to fail" – Benjamin Franklin

Good ole Ben Franklin could not have said it better, planning ahead, without a doubt, is **THE GOLDEN RULE**. If you want to see serious results, then you need to plan each day ahead of time! Now, I do not mean you should necessarily be spending five hours prepping your meals on a Sunday night before a busy week. Sure, you could do that, especially if you enjoy cooking, but it may not be realistic for everyone, and certainly is not a requirement to be successful in this way of eating.

Instead, a good habit to develop would be sitting down each night and planning the meals you would like to eat for the next day using the app. This allows you to foresee issues ahead of time and correct them. For example, if you've plugged in foods you wanted to eat for Monday yet still have 10g of fat to meet, but are out of carbohydrates and protein, you can work to remedy this without feeling put on the spot.

If you had come to this realization at the end of the day on Monday, you would have the choice of munching on a stick of butter or taking a shot of Olive Oil. Seriously. Pure fat is hard to come by in other forms; *don't think I haven't thrown down a few ounces of oily goodness at the end of the night just to hit my numbers.* But, by planning ahead, you can see this issue coming and instead slather some butter on your broccoli at dinner, or add a little extra mayo on your sandwich.

Not planning ahead is like driving cross-country from New York to California without a road map. Sure, eventually you might get to where you want to go, but the journey will probably include unnecessary setbacks and frustrations.

MAKE IT ENJOYABLE

We are not trying to limit any foods, at least not right out of the gate! As I said before, if you love to eat donuts – then that's cool, have the donut, but account for it! When you plan ahead, try plugging that into the app first. Then you can plan the rest of your day *around* that food item and ensure that you get to both hit your macros for the day & enjoy the treat you love to eat.

TAKE BABY STEPS

Trying to hit zero for each macronutrient shown on the MyFitnessPal home screen is a long-term goal; that can be a difficult and even daunting task in the beginning. My suggestion? **Take. Baby. Steps.** You are still learning how to put together meals, plan ahead and navigate the real world with this new lifestyle. On the flipside, if you are finding it an increasingly unobtainable task to hit all of your macros, then we may need to take a different initial approach and focus on one macronutrient at a time and ease into this with a Flexible Eating jump start:

- **Day 1 to 3:** Just track what you normally eat. Don't worry about specific numbers, just learn about your own habits, practice using the app, and get an idea of how much of each macronutrient you typically eat.
- **Day 4 to 6:** Focus on just hitting your protein only since it can be the most difficult (especially for the ladies) to eat in amounts greater than what you were previously used to daily. Make it your goal each day to hit your protein requirement and do your best to not go over on your carbohydrates and fats – but *don't stress out* too much if they aren't entirely perfect.
- **Day 7 to 9:** Hit your protein and carbohydrates. Now that you have a little practice nailing the protein numbers, add in the carbs and keep a watchful eye on the fat intake, but if you go over slightly again no biggie.
- **Day 10:** GO FOR IT! Go all in and hit your macros. Hopefully by this point you have enough practice under your belt to be a

little more comfortable and confident in the process. Now you just need to keep practicing and proficiency will come with time. This is a slower approach, but a slow road to success is infinitely better than a fast burn out.

MACRO DOMINANT FOODS

It's 8:00pm, you have 40g of carbs left before meeting your daily macronutrient requirement. In addition to that, you have perfectly zeroed out your protein and fat *(go you!)*. What's a flexible eater to do?

Well, you have two choices:

1. You can disregard this, and throw caution to the wind that day by having one Boston Kreme Donut which consist of 39g of carbs *(effectively finishing off this macro)*, but also 16g of fat and 3g of protein, which puts you over your daily total for those two macronutrients *(not ideal, please don't do this).*
   or –
2. You can be thoughtful and eat foods that are free or very low in protein and fat – a **macro dominant food.**

A macro dominant food is an item that is fully, or nearly fully, comprised of only one of the three macronutrients and can help us with the aforementioned situation. White Rice would be an example of a food item that is dominant in only carbohydrates – no protein or fat. You can use foods such as this one to help fill gaps in your meals, or to solve situations like the previously outlined Boston Kreme incident or 10g-of-fat dilemma.

PROTEIN DOMINANT FOODS

Use these foods when you need more protein but have already hit or are coming close to your limit on carbs or fat.

Pure Whey Protein Powder: This is great to have on hand. Try to choose brands that have zero carbs and fat, or at least brands that contain very small amounts of them. I personally use and love protein powder from www.Strengthlete.com and my good friend Joe Nissim.

Very Lean Chicken Breast: This contains only about 1.5 grams of fat per serving, and could be even less if you remove any visible trace of yellow chicken fat before cooking it.

Fish: Some fish are very low in fat such as:

- **Atlantic Cod:** 0 carb and .8 grams of fat per serving.
- **Orange Roughy:** 0 carb and .8 grams of fat per serving.
- **Mahi Mahi:** 0 carb and .8 grams of fat per serving.

Egg whites: One egg white provides just a trivial amount of both fat and carbs but 3.6 grams of protein.

Turkey Breast: Roasted turkey breast is just .8 grams of fat per serving and has 0 carbs.

Crabmeat: Alaskan King Crab is just .8 grams of fat per serving and zero carbs. *But remember to skip the dipping butter (it's still pretty good)!*

CARBOHYDRATE DOMINANT FOODS

Use these foods when you need more carbohydrates but have already hit, or are close to, your limit on protein and fat.

While it would definitely be simple to just eat tablespoons of sugar, I'll focus on objectively healthier carb-rich foods.

Fruit: Most fruit is almost fat free and very low in protein:

- **Banana:** A medium size banana has less than .5 grams of fat and only 1.4 grams of protein.
- **Apples:** A large apple has less than a gram of both fat and protein.
- **Blueberries:** A cup has .5 grams of fat and only 1 gram of protein.
- **Strawberries:** A cup of strawberries has less than .5 grams of fat and only 1 gram of protein.
- **Pears:** A large pear has a trivial amount of fat and less than a gram of protein.

Honey: honey is mainly pure sugar, and thus only contains carbohydrates.

Sweet Potatoes: A medium sweet potato has a trivial amount of fat and just 2 grams of protein, but 23 grams of carbohydrates.

Butternut Squash: A cup of roasted butternut squash is virtually fat free and contains less than 2 grams of protein.

Dried Fruit: Dried fruit is a quick way to boost your carb intake in a hurry! Just choose dried fruits with *no added sugar* and ones that are also unsulfured and highly processed, to avoid that here are some of my favorites...

- **Trader Joe's Unsulfured Apricots:** 10 apricots are 50 grams of carbs, 0 grams of fat and only 2 grams of protein, plus 4 grams of fiber.
- **Dried Figs:** 5 dried figs deliver 26 grams of carbs, 0 grams of fat, and 1 gram of protein with 7 grams of fiber.
- **Dried Dates:** This *"as good as candy"* dried fruit contains 31 grams of carbs, 0 grams of fat, 1 gram of protein and 3 grams of fiber per 5 dates.

You can also try virtually anything that is delicious: Licorice *(my go-to!)*, Jelly Beans, Corn Pops!

FAT DOMINANT FOODS

This is one macro group that I never have trouble reaching my daily total for and one that I actually have to work at **NOT** going over on, but I recognize that some flexible eaters may not find it as easy – **especially if you had been stuck in a "low fat" mindset for a long time like the rest of the world thanks to the nifty faulty research I mentioned in that TIME magazine piece earlier.**

At any rate, here are some foods that are rich in healthy fats:

Virgin Olive Oil: 1 tablespoon is 14 grams of fat – and nothing else.

Virgin Coconut Oil: 1 tablespoon similarly contains strictly 14 grams of fat.

Grass-fed Butter: 1 tablespoon is 11.5 grams of fat and has just a trace of carbs and protein.

Nuts: Nuts are high in fat, but do contain some protein and carbs. However, the fat they contain is healthy and by far the *dominant* macro.

- **Almonds:** 10 almonds have 6 grams of fat, 2.4 grams of carbs, and 2.6 grams of protein.
- **Walnuts:** 1 oz contains 18.5 grams of fat, 3.9 grams of carbs, and 4.3 grams of protein.
- **Pecans:** 1 oz delivers 20.4 grams of fat, 4 grams of carbs, and 2.6 grams of protein.

FLEXIBLE EATING TOOLBOX

Here are some tools that I personally use to make my Flexible Eating life easier. While MyFitnessPal's considerable database will help you count your nutrients and macros, it won't be able to weigh the amount you actually eat, or show you how much weight you have lost or gained.

Since I travel a lot I need tools that are sturdy and don't take up too much space. These are *"Jason Ackerman approved"* and if you buy them via Amazon I can't imagine you will be disappointed! Visit www.ownyoureating.com for links to purchase the following items.

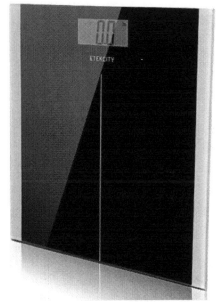

Etekcity Digital Body Weight Bathroom Scale

This scale has a "Step-and-Read" function that will give you immediate readings as soon as you step on the scale. In addition to this it boasts...

- High accuracy – four latest-version high-precision sensors, using technology all the way from Germany!
- Multifunction – Auto-power-off, auto-zero, low battery and overload indication, backlit LCD display.

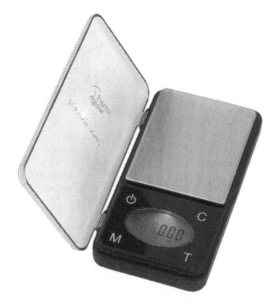

Smart Weigh ZIP600 Ultra Slim Digital Pocket Scale

This Ultra Slim Pocket Scale is lightweight and compact. A flip open cover protects your scale and can be removed to be used as a weighing tray.

- High precision – Manufactured with precision electronic sensors to provide the most accurate measurements. The craftsmanship is of superior quality.
- Maximum capacity of 600 grams and readabilities to 1/10 of a gram, guaranteeing you an accurate and consistent weighing session each time.

This digital food scale is perfect to have in your kitchen to get accurate and fast measurements when Flexible Eating. Wondering what that chicken fillet or piece of Mahi-Mahi really weighs? Just put it on a tray and drop it on the scale!

- Features a newly enlarged weighing platform finished in an elegant chrome and two large buttons that generate an audible click confirmation.
- Precision Tare Button calculates the net weight of your ingredients (it automatically subtracts the weight of any bowl or container!).

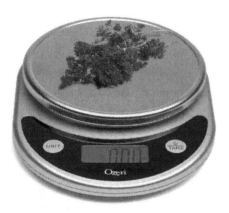

Ozeri Pronto Digital Multifunction Kitchen & Food Scale

Take a break from reading and give yourself a moment or two to digest what you just read. Use this time to think about your eating habits and current relationship with food.

14   This is meant to build on the last question. Are these odd-eating-places planned, or do they happen more spur of the moment? For example, if you eat in the car, do you do this because you are crunched for time or because you feel self-conscious about eating in more of a public place? Hopefully your answer to this will illuminate the type of control eating might have on you (which should ideally be very little).

_____

_____

_____

_____

_____

_____

_____

_____

_____

_____

_____

_____

_____

_____

_____

_____

_____

CHAPTER 17

REBECCA THE INCREDIBLE SHRINKING YOGINI

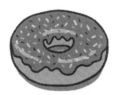

It all started one spring when I went to one of Jason's Flexible Eating seminars. I became interested in attending as a result of my friend Beth losing all of her pregnancy weight working with him – I just had to find out what all this talk was about! I will admit to being skeptical at first, and even after his presentation, I just didn't think all the weighing and measuring was going to work for me. But I was oh so very wrong!

While I was on the fence about the logistical aspects of Flexible Eating; what really struck a chord with me was the discussions about one's own relationship with food – it was honestly something I had never thought about before that day. My whole life I had always been a very fit and athletic person, but then I hit thirty and everything kind of just went downhill. I think I was just doing what most people do, going about my business each day, and over time the weight slowly piled on and I didn't even notice.

Another catalyst for my change was when multiple members of my family lovingly told me that my ass was getting bigger – that was when I realized I really had a problem. My family, of course, are people who love and care about me, so if they're finding the need to tell me this, then I needed to get myself into gear. Jason's seminar, and my family's comments helped me shed a light on and come to terms with my nutritional demons. They gave me the tools and courage to keep emotional eating at bay.

As a nurse, I invest a lot into my patients emotionally which can in turn affect my relationship with food negatively because if they're having a bad day I feel anxious and stressed for them. Couple that with the crazy schedule that comes with the job and it's a recipe for a nutritional disaster. Flexible Eating has helped me find a balance where if I have a bad day it's no big deal at all, I know I can come back and be better on the next. I have control over everything, it's an incredible feeling.

After much hard work, maintaining that balance of macros has given me a lot of success aesthetically. In the past I would do so much cardio and practice Yoga to burn calories at **THOSE** moments, but not think about what I was doing to achieve my goals during the other 23 hours of the day. Now I think a lot about what I'm putting into my body and I can honestly tell you that there's no way I was eating this much protein before – it's still a challenge some days! However, the dramatic changes I've seen in my body composition are well worth the struggle.

Quite simply, it's all about the nutrition.

Not only has Flexible Eating helped me build the body that I want, but it has also helped relieve the chronic back pain I was suffering from. Of course, losing 50 lbs. of body weight helps, but I came to realize that some of the foods I was eating previously were also contributing to the pain. Call me crazy, but when I would eat cheese it would affect my intestines in such a way that caused back pain. I never really put two and two together before to make the connection.

But, with that pain gone, hitting postures in yoga has become so much easier and pleasurable. I can proudly say I can hold handstands and chin balances now where in the past those poses would have been too difficult. People in my class even joke that I'm the incredible shrinking woman!

My advice for anyone looking for a change in their lifestyle is to give Flexible Eating a shot. When you do, try not to let yourself become overwhelmed and instead embrace the process of changing your mindset towards nutrition – once I did that everything became so incredibly easy. You're going to learn so much about yourself and gain a lot of perspective and guidance that will help you achieve your goals.

Most importantly – like me – you will reestablish a healthier relationship with food that is sustainable in the long term. It's truly empowering to know I can look how I want, and live the lifestyle I want, all by eating the foods I want!

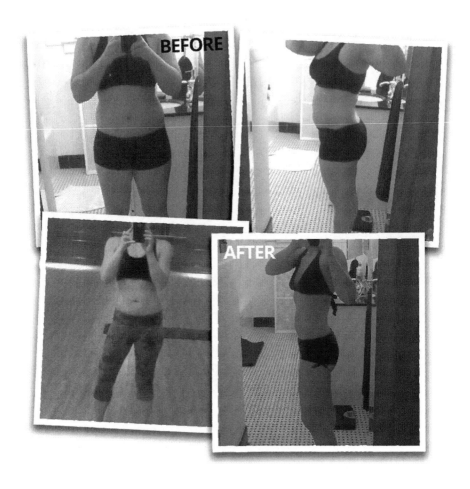

CHAPTER 18

KEEPING IT SUSTAINABLE

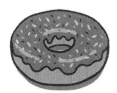

Conventional wisdom would have you believe that to achieve your goals you must:

1. "Eat Less" – often at an extreme or even dangerous caloric deficit.
2. Endure the process for an arbitrary amount of time i.e. 30 / 60 / or 90 days for a miracle to happen. This isn't realistic because life still happens while you are going through the process. Have you ever seen those "post-show" pics of the crazy food people inhale after months of deprivation? That's what happens when you combine a time constraint with a miserable diet. As soon as your "time" is up you essentially become a human garbage disposal, throwing away months of literal blood, sweat, tears, and hours of training by binging on Dunkin' Donuts or S'mores Pop-Tarts. Worth it? Of course not! Especially when you take into account that you could've

been enjoying these things in *reasonable amounts* this whole time, all the while getting the same (if not better) results!

3. Restricting or eliminating foods that you actually enjoy to eat and replacing them with ultra-low-cal-low-taste-low-everything alternatives. I mean sure, cut down to 500 calories a day and you'll drop weight like nothing; but this is neither healthy, nor sustainable, nor likely to last any substantial amount of time. This is what people are usually referring to with the term "Yo-Yoing" – your weight shooting up and down like that damn toy. But that's not the only thing to be concerned about – what about the effect all that up 'n' down has on your brain, organs, physical performance and mood? Why would you purposely endure that hell when you have the perfect solution? Eat what you want to fill your macronutrient balances and then go out and kick some ass.

Counting your macronutrients and utilizing MyFitnessPal certainly has its challenges, but there are *plenty* of steps you can take to keep this lifestyle sustainable as you build new habits and establish a lifelong relationship with food that is stronger and more sensible. Let's address some ways to troubleshoot some common struggles...

DINING OUT

Tracking your macronutrients can become tricky when dining out. Tricky, but not impossible – I do it on a weekly basis. Here is what I recommend you do to avoid exceeding your macronutrients when you're at the mercy of a restaurant, or just someone else's kitchen.

◉ **When your foods are in the app:** In a perfect world, you would have advance notice of when and where you will be dining out. This way, you can pick what you plan to eat ahead of time and log that into the app. Then, you can have what you want to eat and simply plan the rest of your day (and your remaining macronutrients). But, we're not in an ideal world, so let's look at what will likely happen… Friday night rolls around and you and your special someone usually meet for dinner after work, at the restaurant where you met *(*heart flutter*)*. Luckily, MyFitnessPal has an extensive database for most popular places to eat. You can still hit up their online menu and choose a meal that appropriately suits your macro-needs. Easy!

- **When your foods are not in the app:** These days, most mainstream places will have the nutritional content for their menu items listed on their website, and you can manually enter these into MyFitnessPal in the case that it is not already in the database. If you can't find anything online, you can always ask your waiter if they have anything available, like a printed-out nutritional pamphlet, that you could look through. If you're dining at a local, smaller joint, and don't have any access to nutritional info, you can just try your best to log your meal based on similar foods in the app and what you have had at other places. In this scenario, the simpler you keep your order, the easier hitting your macros on point will be for you.

- For instance, if you order a steak, the protein and fat content will generally be the same wherever you decide to eat. The difference, though, will be the serving size. So, make sure to plug this into the app to ensure precision and to create a reference point for future situations. The same goes for when ordering a side of vegetables; log the portion amount of each item and enjoy! Really, I'm serious. Don't glaze over this last point; because enjoying the times you go out is just as important and is what makes for a happy mind *and* belly.

- **When your destination is unknown:** You may not always be afforded the luxury of knowing where (and when) you will end up eating – this is especially true for those who travel a lot. In these situations, I recommend just trying to do your best to eat a large amount of proteins throughout the day, and saving your fats & carbohydrates for the later hours. This is because it is oftentimes difficult to go out to eat and get a substantial amount of protein on the road, but the other two macronutrients can be easily satisfied in one meal *(hello, dessert!)*. **For example:** if you are someone who needs 150g of protein a day I would leave something like approximately 30 to 50g of protein for dinner and a substantial amount of fat & carbohydrates, relative to the amount of food you typically eat.

A Typical Question: Will eating out too often ruin my Flexible Eating plan?

Well, if you're diligent about tracking what you eat on the regular, then there's no reason eating out will hinder your overall progress. But, as we discussed above, it does make Flexible Eating a bit more complicated than it needs to be.

While eating out won't necessarily harm your Flexible-Eating-Flow, I do see a few health related issues with it, that may end up interfering with your *overall* health.

1. With eating out there is so much that is out of your control in the way of ingredient qualities, reasonable portion sizes, amount of salt used – all of which can be challenging in and of themselves. What's more, when you eat out you usually don't *want* this kind of control, the whole idea is to kick back, relax, have a good time and not have to do a mountain of dishes after. You don't go out to get a burger wrapped in a collard leaf and a side of steamed carrots.

2. Another problem I see with eating out? People also tend to underestimate the calorie count on servings. If you eat out a lot and aren't diligent about tracking your numbers, those extra three bites of pasta **do** really throw off your daily accountability. It sucks I know; but bites count. Everything really

does need to be accounted for to make results happen, and sometimes you have to throw away half of that red velvet cheesecake.

I think eating out in moderation is the best course of action. The majority of what you eat should be within your control – but you also need to give yourself the freedom and fun of eating out, or else this will just become another restrictive diet that ultimately fails. Don't turn Flexible Eating into something it isn't; you are supposed to eat and do the things that make you happy!

Flexible Eating is a way to eat for life that allows for living. So go out there and do just that.

Here's a great portion size reference to consult when you are unsure of how much you are eating.

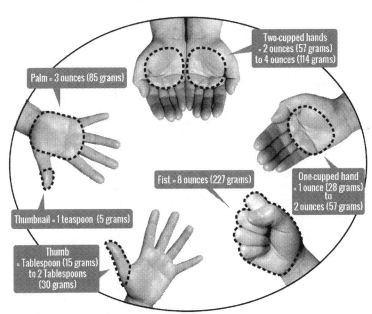

Note: Measurements may vary depending on hand size.

[Figure 18.1]

Now, let's talk about something a little different than the ole hum-drum Friday night date night: eating out for *special* occasions.

- **Special Events:** First, it is important that you define "special event" realistically and reasonably. Going out to the bar every Friday night is not a special event that justifies going completely off the rails. I'm talking about weddings, reunions, anniversaries, birthday parties, baby showers, things like that. My point here is that you shouldn't go crazy at them, but you don't need to be the weirdo with a scale at the table measuring out individual potato chips. If you are calculating correctly, you shouldn't even feel the need to go crazy in the first place. Your brain and body are getting their needs met. Graze throughout the day and leave a substantial number of macros (similar to the ones you would allot in the above Destination Unknown scenario). Log what you eat, monitor the app to make sure you do not go overboard, but also remember to enjoy yourself. The next day can always be better.

- **Vacations:** The more damage you do the longer it will take to reverse it. That being said **ENJOY YOURSELF**. If you are on a cruise, tropical get away, or even out of town for a week you no doubt paid a pretty penny for the experience. I expect you to relax, get the full value of the trip and take a vacation from *everything* in your daily life including macronutrients & MyFitnessPal. That will all be waiting for you when you return, believe me. But, that being said, I don't recommend doing this more than once or twice a year.

ALCOHOL

Nutrient dense foods will ultimately be the heroes to help us reach our goals, but I know we all love to go out with friends at the end of a long work week and kick back with a few beers or a bottle of wine. It is important to note that alcoholic beverages have *minimal nutritional value*. If you are going to indulge you need to take a few things into consideration:

1. **"But there's only 3g of carbs?!":** Most beer companies do not account for all of the macronutrients in their product labelling. A Michelob Ultra may boast to only contain 3g of carbohydrates per serving and **ONLY** 100 calories. But, we know better – if you think back to *Chapter 6 – Flexible Eating, Defined* – 1g of carbohydrate equates to 4 calories. So, 3g x 4 = 12 calories. So where are the other 88 unaccounted for calories coming from?

2. **Sugar Alcohol:** Those extra calories are coming from sugar alcohol, and the beer companies are not taking it into consideration when pushing their product. This means that having four beers with your pals could give you an excess of 100 carbs instead, of the 12 you might have thought you were taking in.

3. **Tracking:** To take into account the carbohydrates provided by the Sugar Alcohol you simply need to divide the total calories in the drink by 4. **In the case of beer, it would be:** 100 (calories) / 4 (calories per 1 gram of carb) = 25g of carbs total. This number, 25g, is what you would track in MyFitnessPal. The same method would be used for wine. Divide the number of calories per serving by 4.

When you look at each beer as costing you 25g of carbohydrates instead of 3g, it puts a little more perspective on how alcohol can derail your day (or even your week!) if you seriously indulge. If you absolutely want to have those four beers, that's okay; log them in the app first and then plan the rest of your day around it. You just might be eating a lot of naked sandwiches that day. Understand where and how alcohol fits into your life, just try not to overdo it.

All of this is to say that I cannot emphasize enough that you **DO NOT** need to be extremely restrictive with your eating. No one wants to be that guy or gal at a party who is "not allowed" to have cake. It's not fun being around them and it's *certainly* not fun actually being them. In the end it all comes down to this: **ENJOY YOURSELF - BUT BE SMART ABOUT IT**. There is no reason that enjoyment has to go hand in hand with uninhibited binging. With continued practice you will find a groove that allows you to operate on cruise control, while you achieve your goals. It gets easier, I promise.

Take a break from reading and give yourself a moment or two to digest what you just read. Use this time to think about your eating habits and current relationship with food.

15   Recount your experience the last time you went on a diet. Go into detail about why you pursued the diet, how long it lasted, results you saw, what happened over time... I want to know everything!

_____

_____

_____

_____

_____

_____

_____

_____

_____

_____

_____

_____

_____

_____

_____

_____

_____

_____

_____

_____

16   Did this diet "work?" If not, can you nail down the reasons why?

CHAPTER 19

HOWIE'S STORY: DRINK BEER & LOSE WEIGHT

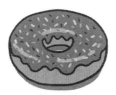

Jason and I have been good friends since attending the University at Albany (SUNY Albany) in Albany, New York some twenty plus years ago. I remember *(well...to the extent that copious amounts of alcohol consumption will allow)* those days and the memories we created together at the Long Branch Tavern fondly – especially free beer Tuesday nights. Even then, aside from the drinking, Jason could be considered the "fitness guy." He has always had that passion for exercising and was always on some sort of dietary kick. As for myself, well, now I'm a different story as I'm more of your typical "normal guy" who works a regular nine to five job while raising two wonderful children alongside my beautiful wife Jen. Having six pack abs or being healthy for a guy like me meant I would have to spend endless hours exercising and eating foods I hate or even worse give up beer, right?

Well, for a long time I thought that was the case. I have never really been a person that enjoys to exercise – heck I do not even have a gym membership that I pay for, but do not use. I am just completely off the fitness industries grid. To be even more honest, before working directly with Jason, making my nutrition and health were not on the forefront of my mind. I think that's a quality I share with many parents out there who work a full-time job most days of the week and on others spend the majority of the time taking care of the kids. It can be a struggle to take care of yourself when you're constantly taking care of someone else. That was my general thought process and it took me some time to realize that all I was doing was making excuses.

My wife Jen is simply amazing. She has always had a better handle on her health than I did by making the time to go to Spin or some other group exercise class most days of the week. Not only has she blessed me with two beautiful children, but she was also the catalyst that prompted me to start my Flexible Eating journey. Jen had scheduled a phone consultation with Jason to discuss starting a macro plan and I sat in on the tail end of the conversation – it intrigued me and more importantly got the wheels in my head turning. You see, Jen and I love each other dearly, but I had felt for some time that she was not happy with the lifestyle I was living. She never said so directly and it's entirely possible that I was projecting my own feelings about myself onto her because deep down I was not happy with my health. Either way, I needed to change and was ready to pursue one.

The week following that phone call, Jen and I attended one of Jason's Flexible Eating seminars to spend some time with him, learn more information, and immerse ourselves in the process. The fact that we were going to take control of our nutrition together as a family made the whole adventure into macros, MyFitnessPal, and watching Jason's half naked YouTube videos super easy. Flashforward from then to now and the results I have achieved are fantastic. I still do not exercise at all, eat way more food, and have lost a grand total of 45 lbs. – I could not be happier with the progress!

Solely through Flexible Eating I am able to manage my body weight and still eat and drink the things that make me happy such as beer. Speaking of beer, I am a bit of a connoisseur of the bubbly, hops filled beverage. Prior to Flexible Eating, I would drink up to six beers after putting the kids to bed – most parents out there undoubtedly understand the need. Now I'm not a beer snob by any means, but if I am able to I prefer to buy specialty beers that can sometimes contain up to 200 calories per bottle. These beers are expensive in regards to my daily macro bank account costing me 50g of carbohydrates each. That might be enough to deter most people from indulging in an iced cold brewski, but for me therein lies the change – I plan ahead to use those 50g of carbs for my beer – doing that gives me peace of mind which in turn helps me to maintain a level of consistency. All of those pieces to the puzzle help me to live a realistic and sustainable lifestyle that yields astonishing results.

The flexibility of Jason's Flexible Eating method is absolutely remarkable in that it can mold into whatever the user needs. Even if you find it challenging to make time to workout at a gym or just plain old do not like exercising; you can still take over the reins of your health, guide it in a new direction, and have the body you have always wanted. You can eat anything you want as long as you are diligent in your tracking. My biggest piece of advice to others would be to actually use the tools that have been provided to you by Jason to determine your food choices for each day. Take the time to make a plan using his wisdom because that will be the easiest way to develop a level of consistency.

I couldn't be happier with what I have achieved through Flexible Eating. My wife is more attracted to me *(you know what they say: happy wife, happy life)*, I feel confident in my own skin because I look better, and I lost 45 lbs. while drinking beer and not exercising. Most importantly, I have learned a system that I can continue to use on a daily basis for the rest of my life: Flexible Eating.

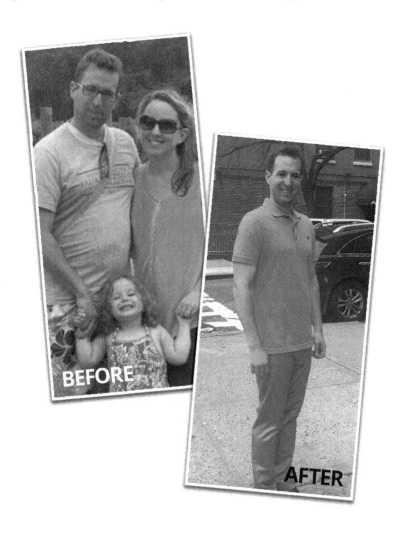

CHAPTER 20

TWEAKING 'N' REVERSE DIETING

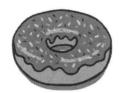

At some point it will become necessary to tweak your numbers. This only needs to be done when your body reaches a plateau, but you still have ways to go in reaching your goals. Just because you have these numbers does not necessarily mean they will perfectly lead you to the ultimate success. There are several lifestyle factors we need to take into consideration on why the scale is not moving in the desired direction before tweaking your numbers such as:

1. Work, family, and other life stresses.
2. Lack of sleep.
3. Your level of Consistency.

SLEEP, STRESS AND CORTISOL

It is never a good idea to obsess over the scale daily and to beat yourself up when the numbers you want to see aren't there to greet you each morning. In that scenario, if the number isn't going the direction you want it to, it would instead be better for you to ask yourself **"do I have all of my bases covered?"** To dive deeper into that question: do you have your sleep schedule in check? Are you letting the little things in life like your job, school papers that you've been procrastinating on starting, or fights with your special someone stress you out all the time? Yes, all of those situations are *the little things* your **health** is the big thing, so let's focus on it first by starting with a little shut-eye – we will be able to think a little more clearly on everything after a good night's sleep.

Sleep is one of those things that you literally just can't live without. Unfortunately, many try to skate by with caffeine coursing through their veins and minimal pillow time. You may be able to fool everyone else with all the energy you put on display, but you can't fool your closest friend – your body. Sleep is that special time where important recovery work happens; your body repairs muscles, soothes aches 'n' pains and all of the other bodily systems have time to rejuvenate.

Depriving yourself of that important quality time spent in dream land is going to increase your chances of feeling lethargic, run-down and maybe even a little cranky. What's worse is that even though you may adamantly claim that you can survive on five hours of sleep each night, your body is stressed out (and tired!) and that's due to a hormone called **Cortisol**. As your body's number one stress hormone, cortisol, is released into the bloodstream when you are **emotionally** or **physically stressed**.

It's cortisol's job to deal with stress within the body by releasing large amounts of glucose into the bloodstream when you're in a fight or flight (stressful) situation. The problems are **a.)** you don't need fast acting energy, but instead more **zZz** and **b.)** that the energy provided by glucose is taken from protein stores within the liver (which is supposed to be used for other things such as nervous system function!). This is through a process called gluconeogenesis (that we discussed in greater detail in *Chapter 7 – Building Blocks*), where protein is converted into fast acting energy to use in stressful (and intense) situations: CrossFit workouts, running from a bear, or lack of sleep. In a normal situation i.e. post-exercise, your body would use elevated blood sugar levels, along with insulin, to help shuttle protein back into muscles for recovery.

In our scenario, protein is not being brought back to muscle tissue because they're still full due to protein being taken from the liver in the first place. The glucose currently in the bloodstream will eventually be stored as fat because there's nowhere else for it to go. Why can't it just go back to the liver? Because that backup storage center is tapped into only *after* muscles are replenished and we cannot skip the order of operations here.

This is a pretty big deal! Elevated cortisol levels and the bodily stress that comes with it, slows down, or even stops you from reaching your goals. If you want to look better naked, lose weight and perform well then you need to get your sleep schedule in order **AND** get your stress levels managed. Otherwise, even if you hit your daily macronutrients perfectly and exercise intelligently, the lack of sleep and abundance of stress will still be too much for your body to handle and it will prioritize those regulations over burning fat.

CONSISTENCY

Once you have your sleep schedule and stress levels in check, the next most important thing I want to know before we tweak your macros is whether or not you are hitting your numbers? If you are not consistently consuming all of your daily macronutrients we shouldn't be altering your numbers. If you're not putting in the effort needed; we would likely be lowering or raising your numbers only to find the same lack of results. You need to successfully hit your numbers for at least seven days (in a row, if that wasn't obvious) before you consider making any adjustments.

Your metabolism is going to play a big role in overcoming plateaus. Imagine you're doing an oil change on your car. You're not taking out 100% of the old oil and replacing it with the new. It takes some time to cycle through the old stuff! Your metabolism is just like this; it is improving slowly. The changes made are gradual, not all at once. Over time, your body might reach a sort of equilibrium state in which case a slight tweak can be useful to rev the macro-engine again.

INSTITUTING CHANGES

When tweaking your numbers, it is important that the changes you make are not drastic ones. I recommend no more than a 5% decrease or increase in carbohydrates and fats. Make no changes to protein since that is based off your goal lean body mass. You are going to have to be a guinea pig and test different macronutrient counts out to see what works for you.

Whatever it is that you decide upon, please do not forget that if you are not consistently hitting your numbers then there is no way we can pass a judgement on whether or not the numbers are optimal for you. That would be like buying a gym membership, never going, and then blaming the gym for when you inexplicably only get chubbier and more out of shape.

If you are stuck 5 to 10 lbs. away from your goal, then you more than likely need to decrease your numbers. If you are within 5 lbs. of your goal weight, then consider adding more food. If you know you have a special event coming up, then wait until after to make any tweaks to your numbers.

REFEED DAYS

A refeed day is also another good strategy to stoke the flames of your metabolism again as it can help to reboot a hormone called Leptin. Leptin, otherwise known as the "satiety hormone," aids in regulating energy balance by inhibiting hunger. When you lose a good deal of excess body fat weight you may experience a drop in levels of leptin circulating in the bloodstream. This drop can cause a reversible decrease in thyroid activity and energy expenditure in skeletal muscle. If a person loses weight below their natural body fat set point, this can lead to lower basal metabolic rate than a person of the same weight that is naturally that weight.

This homeostatic response is meant to reduce energy expenditure and weight gain as a result of fat cells being shrunken below normal size. A refeed day can help to reverse this response by providing an overabundance of calories that the body is currently not used to.

Importantly, though, is that when conducting a refeed day, we still want to have approximately the same number of calories, and just vary the number of macros. Keep the same amount of protein, but eat more carbohydrates and less fat than you are used to on a typical day. The first thing to do is take away some fat calories. Let's say you consume 68g of fat in a day, we will divide that by 2 and our new total for the day will be 34g. This means that we will be decreasing fat intake by 306 calories. So, we just want to allocate those calories to our carbohydrates. We can figure this out by dividing 306 by 4, meaning that you should eat an additional 77g of carbohydrates. Thus, we now have the same daily calories, but with a different ratio of macronutrients. I would only recommend doing this when your overall numbers are pretty low.

REVERSE DIETING

Another strategy for breaking through plateaus is reverse dieting. Reverse dieting is where we go the other direction and add more food (or macronutrients) as opposed to taking them away. You would utilize this method if you are currently at your goal weight, very close to it, are hungry all the time, or notice your performance in the gym decreasing. If and only if you are consistently hitting your numbers; we can add more food and see how your body will respond. Refer to **Figure 19.1** for extra guidance on whether or not you are truly plateauing and if you should change your numbers.

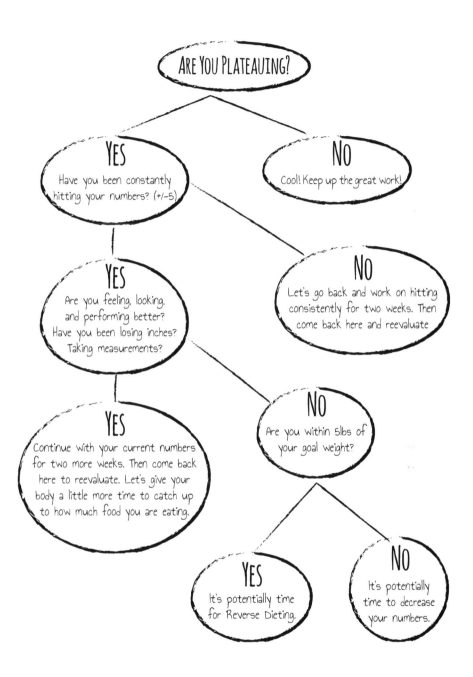

[Figure 19.1]

Take a break from reading and give yourself a moment or two to digest what you just read. Use this time to think about your eating habits and current relationship with food.

17   If the diet you were on previously **DID** work, what happened in the days following the end of the diet? Were you able to keep your results?

_____

_____

_____

_____

_____

_____

_____

_____

_____

_____

_____

_____

_____

_____

_____

_____

_____

_____

_____

_____

_____

_____

CHAPTER 21

PAGING NURSE LAUREN

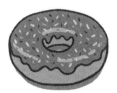

Prior to my pregnancy, I never really had to worry too much about food or my body weight. I had a great routine, going to CrossFit classes most days of the week, and running here and there for a little extra cardio. My diet was about 75% Paleo during the week and then the weekends would turn into "cheat days" filled with waffles, pizza, and Oreos – okay I'll admit to having a bit of a sweet tooth!

You know I just didn't really think about the amount of food I was eating; since I wasn't gaining weight there was no concern. That all changed drastically though when I became pregnant with my son Jude. I soon found out that pregnancy is a funny thing in a sense where your body will ask for foods you would normally avoid. For example: I never drank milk in the past, but had it throughout my entire pregnancy. I would also eat tons of beef stew, hamburgers, meatloaf and pot roast – my body must have been craving all the iron those foods provide.

I was definitely eating more food than I normally would. Luckily, I work as a pediatric nurse, so I was well aware of the recommended guidelines for healthy pregnancy weight gain – which is 300 extra calories while pregnant and another 200 while nursing. Doing that, I increased in body weight from 140 lbs. to 175 lbs. which was a very reasonable increase.

My advice for future moms out there is that when your body asks for something, listen to it, but be sensible. When I'm at work I see it all the time, women thinking they have a free pass to binge eat because they are expecting. They end up putting on 70 to 100 lbs. of excess weight and it definitely effects their health negatively. The goal should be to support healthy weight gain and the baby with your eating, and that's it. Everyone is definitely going to be different in what they need, but just don't go crazy about it. The public in general has a big misconception about eating and pregnancy, but your doctor will tell you the truth – there is no free pass.

When I eventually had Jude, I soon realized that the first six months were going to be incredibly difficult. I was sleeping very little, eating, waking up all hours of the night, eating, nursing, eating, and then eating again because I was starving! After all, I was sharing my body's nutrients with Jude – it was exhausting. I know that I, and I'm sure many other moms out there do as well, ended up putting my personal health on the back burner for my baby.

I'm happy to say though that there will come a point when it's time to focus on **YOU** again. For me it was about nine months after giving birth when Jude wasn't nursing anymore. I felt that I could finally have a moment or two of clarity and give myself the attention my body needed. I started my old routine right back up again, taking classes at Albany CrossFit, and made an effort to eat clean. The only problem was that the weight was just not coming off!

For some women the weight just melts away after they have their baby, but I was stuck. I had seen so many people raving about Flexible Eating on Facebook and decided to give it a shot. Once I had my own macro numbers,

I soon realized that what my body needed now was much different from what it needed close to a year earlier. I needed to pay special attention to my diet and now I had the control to really dial in my nutrition.

Every day was an opportunity to practice and I eventually figured out a system and everything became quite easy. Within the first few weeks, I had lost a few pounds and I started to feel better about myself. Really the main challenge was finding the balance around managing my macros – and – taking care of Jude. I make it a point each night to plan ahead and having the ability to adjust that plan has been key. Sometimes I might have to go to the gym later than I expected and it's tough to bring myself to cook a meal when I get home. I just remind myself, the math is already done and I'm doing this for me. I always feel better about making the effort and put together something quick and easy like stir fry.

About a month into my Flexible Eating journey I went on vacation to Mexico with my husband Peter and Jude. I decided to not worry about the macros, they would be there waiting for me when I returned from vacation – which was a huge relief because I really just wanted to chill out and finally relax. I was also **THRILLED** to find my pre-pregnancy bikinis and shorts all fit. The surprises just kept coming and upon returning home I discovered that I had not gained any extra weight and had a plan that I could get right back into. The app and the numbers never go away as long as I am willing to put in the effort.

The improvements I have made on the scale and in the gym have also reaffirmed that the struggles are worth it! Since I began to eat flexibly, I have dropped 12 lbs. and ended up doing my very first pull-up! Other changes in my performance have included a 37 lbs. personal record on my deadlift which is now 187 lbs. and a 15 lbs. improvement on my clean and jerk at 100 lbs. It's pretty darn satisfying to see everything in my fitness improving. I feel like my body is fuelled now to do the things I want to do.

My main piece of advice to someone just starting out would be that mastery does not come right away. You have to give yourself time and learn how to count your macros. That also includes having the patience to wait for the results – things don't just happen overnight. You just need to stick with it and amazing things will happen. Oh, and you have to plan, plan, plan ahead! Have your fridge stocked with protein and know what you are going to eat ahead of time.

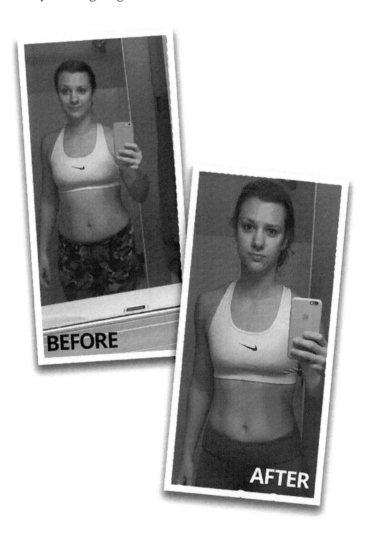

CHAPTER 22

CUTTING WEIGHT FOR SPORT

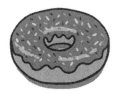

I know some of you readers are probably involved in a sport that requires you to be a certain weight for competition. This chapter is really just for you. If you are just the average Joe looking to drop a couple of pounds then by all means please read on for educational purposes, but be aware I do not recommend you follow any of these practices. The methods we are using are to achieve goals other than losing weight to maintain a healthy lifestyle. This isn't to say I will be suggesting any unhealthy or damaging practices, but they do not align with **YOUR** goals (if you are that average Joe).

Now, let's get down to it. The main rule with participating in a weight class sport is making the clear distinction between where you would *like* to be vs. where you *need* to be:

- **Where you would like to be:** The more attuned you are with your body and with the sport, the better you will be able to gauge the weight you like to perform at. Most athletes will know where they feel the best and do well.

○ **Where you need to be:** Where you would like to be sometimes is at odds with where you need to be in order to *win*. Winning is the ultimate goal in sports and it will change based on the competitors who show up.

○ In wrestling, I always trained a few pounds heavier leading up to the day of the meet. It helped me keep my strength and energy. I would cut down before weigh-ins – which in wrestling was typically the day before the match. The time after that was then spent refueling. So, it happened that when I actually wrestled, I was much heavier than what I weighed in at. It helped to be the heavier guy in the weight class because it, obviously, gave me a little bit of an advantage over someone who was smaller and lighter.

That might not always be the case in other sports. In weightlifting for example, you weigh-in the same day you compete. It is very important to make sure you have the energy to lift heavy weights and you may not even have the advantage by being the heavier competitor. For example, if two athletes end a competition lifting a 200 kg total whoever was *lighter* would be decided as the winner.

We need to make sure things are done in a healthy and safe way when undergoing a longer cut. I recently went through the process with one of my now longtime clients, Robert. He was originally a CrossFitter, but around the time he started Flexible Eating, he became especially interested in participating in his first weightlifting meet.

Both myself and Robert were excited to test out a new method of Flexible Eating to suit this, so we took the thing for a spin! We picked a local meet for him to sign up for and his training became a tag team effort between myself and the *Own Your Eating's* co-author James

McDermott, who is also an experienced weightlifting coach. I crunched the macro numbers and James provided the weekly programming.

When Robert started he weighed 178 lbs. which would put him in the 85 kg (169.422 lbs. to 187 lbs.) weight class for his new sport. His goal weight was 160 lbs. Dropping 18 lbs. would put Robert in a new weight class of 77 kg (151.822 to 169.4 lbs.). We had a good amount of time until his competition, about two months, so we decided to go for it!

Most CrossFit guys carry a little bit of extra weight, but I knew we could make interesting things happen with Robert. With two months of training to fine tune his skills; and 18 lbs. to lose we needed to make sure all of our ducks were in a row.

I met with Robert daily via Skype to help him plan. Luckily, he is a by-the-numbers, very meticulous type of guy and took our experiment seriously. It added another level of focus to his overall training that he admitted he lacked before.

Robert, was a creature of habit and ate relatively the same foods each day, which made using the MyFitnessPal app and consistently hitting his numbers easier for him. To maintain his strength during training and leading up to the meet, we kept his protein higher than normal at 150g – instead of 144g which would normally be 90% of his goal weight. As seen in **Table 21.1**, Robert's carbs would slowly decrease by 5g for the first five weeks and then 10g for the last three. Fat was reduced in a similar fashion: 1g each week for the first five, and then 2g the last three weeks.

When the big day arrived Robert weighed in well within the 77 kg weight class at 74 kg (162.8 lbs.) – just 2.8 lbs. away from his overall goal weight! He had an incredible day, setting a five-pound personal record snatch at 170 lbs., and a fifteen-pound personal record clean and jerk of 220 lbs., and successfully completed 5 of 6 lifting attempts to place 8th in the weight class – not too shabby for a first time outing!

Needless to say, it was an awesome first time experience for Robert and I am happy to report that besides the expected nerves, he had a tremendous amount of energy all day. His body had slowly adapted over the previous eight weeks to use the food he ate more efficiently. Though he had lost about 16 lbs., he wasn't depleted. The first half of this experiment was a success…but we were not done yet!

Weeks	Daily Macronutrients (Cutting Weight)
One	**Calories:** 2,012 **Protein:** 150g | **Carbs:** 195g | **Fat:** 68g * Keep Protein high to maintain strength during the cut.
Two	**Calories:** 1,980 | **Protein:** 150g | **Carbs:** 190g | **Fat:** 67g
Three	**Calories:** 1,954 | **Protein:** 150g | **Carbs:** 185g | **Fat:** 66g
Four	**Calories:** 1,925 | **Protein:** 150g | **Carbs:** 180g | **Fat:** 65g
Five	**Calories:** 1,896 | **Protein:** 150g | **Carbs:** 175g | **Fat:** 64g
Six	**Calories:** 1,838 | **Protein:** 150g | **Carbs:** 170g | **Fat:** 62g
Seven	**Calories:** 1,780 | **Protein:** 150g | **Carbs:** 160g | **Fat:** 60g
Eight	**Calories:** 1,722 | **Protein:** 150g | **Carbs:** 150g | **Fat:** 58g

[Table 21.1]

This is just one example of how you could go about cutting for a meet and one that we have found success with. The point is to decrease macros slowly to give your body time to adjust and kick into a new gear each week. It's certainly not perfect and you may be at a point in your Flexible Eating journey where your cut looks very different. It's important to work with a coach if you're in doubt.

The key is taking things slow and steady to make sure you maintain maximum strength while losing at a moderate pace on the scale. You will feel and perform better this way, as opposed to making a drastic change to your diet one or two weeks out. We highly recommend some trial and error prior to diving into this way of eating before competition.

Try the cut when you have no big events on the calendar, to see if it would work for you.

Directly after competition is a crucial period. The meet is over, and now it's time to return to a *normal* eating regime. It is really important to ease back into normal numbers slowly; if you just jump right back to your original, higher, numbers, you risk putting on a lot of excess fat. Your body is no longer used to that amount of food. Its ability to efficiently process the higher quantity of nutrients will be a little off, so we need to account for that.

Weeks	Daily Macronutrients (Reverse Dieting)
One	**Calories:** 1,780 | **Protein:** 150g | **Carbs:** 160g | **Fat:** 60g
Two	**Calories:** 1,896 | **Protein:** 150g | **Carbs:** 180g | **Fat:** 64g
Three	**Calories:** 1,954 | **Protein:** 150g | **Carbs:** 190g | **Fat:** 66g
Four	**Calories:** 2,012 | **Protein:** 150g | **Carbs:** 200g | **Fat:** 68g
Five	**Calories:** 2,088 | **Protein:** 150g | **Carbs:** 210g | **Fat:** 72g
Six	**Calories:** 2,164 | **Protein:** 150g | **Carbs:** 220g | **Fat:** 76g
Seven	**Calories:** 2,240 | **Protein:** 150g | **Carbs:** 230g | **Fat:** 80g
Eight	**Calories:** 2,316 | **Protein:** 150g | **Carbs:** 240g | **Fat:** 84g

[Table 21.2]

After a competition your first instinct is going to be to binge on all sorts of food and celebrate – but don't! Your goals as an athlete are hopefully worth more to you than that. Robert was a perfect example and recognized that his job was not yet done. He was readily prepared to keep following our prescription once the competition was over. I was there to give Robert the support he needed and made sure he got back on track right away. As seen in **Table 21.2**, through reverse dieting we gradually increased his macros back to his starting point, and where we even eventually surpassed his starting numbers.

The end results were amazing! Robert is now in a new weight class, and we were able to get him there safely. He's eating more food daily than before, which certainly gives him more energy and helps with his weightlifting overall. We can owe all of this success to the fact that we were deliberate in creating and sticking to his numbers easing him off a cut.

What I hope you get from this is that cutting weight is a very sensitive operation.

Personal health is always our first priority. There are tons of "dirtier" practices out there that will get you the same weight come weigh-in day (and many of which I have performed in the past – such as complete starvation). But at what cost are you getting those results? I remember back in my wrestling days I resorted to eating ice cubes to keep my sanity. I hope it goes without saying, that this is **not** healthy and **I do not recommend** any other methods than what is listed above.

Basically, keep it clean, with real food. Adjusting your numbers correctly will be the key to not only arriving at where you want or need to be, but maintaining health and your level of performance – especially at competition time, when it really matters.

Take a break from reading and give yourself a moment or two to digest what you just read. Use this time to think about your eating habits and current relationship with food.

18   What are the major influences on what, when, and how you eat? Time, family, friends, special occasions?

_____

_____

_____

_____

_____

_____

_____

_____

_____

_____

_____

_____

_____

_____

_____

_____

_____

_____

_____

_____

_____

19 Are these influences keeping you from being happy and reaching your goals? Are you willing to address them? Are you willing to sit down with your friends and family to tell them how you feel?

CHAPTER 23

FOLEY, CHRIS FOLEY... SHAKEN NOT STIRRED

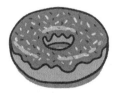

When I was younger my relationship with food was deeply tied into wrestling. The food I was putting into my mouth was always an issue, especially when I was trying to cut weight. I just didn't understand how to maintain a solid healthy body weight and lacked any sort of guidance on how to do so – if only I knew about Flexible Eating back then.

Cut, cut, cut, and then binge, binge, binge – that was the extent of the knowledge within the sport. In addition to that, before a competition I would sit in the sauna wearing a rubber suit, spit into cups (gross I know!), and starve myself to make weight. After weigh-ins, it was like a holiday, a celebration of the food that I had been missing throughout the weeks.

Being a young guy I was pretty resilient and my body could handle all the ups and downs wrestling demanded of my diet. The real problem came when I grew older, stopped wrestling, but continued my bad eating habits – they certainly caught up with me. Once my wrestling career was over I just went nuts all the time eating whatever I wanted and whenever I wanted it. The weight gain was slow and I didn't notice it until one day I looked at myself in the mirror and thought "**WOW!** I look like I'm wearing a fat suit!" It was a horrifying realization that I had let myself go so badly and the kick in the butt I needed to make a change.

Although I wanted to make swift changes to my lifestyle, I still lacked guidance and after searching around the internet for options, I eventually settled on giving the Atkins diet a shot. In the beginning it was cool to see the scale slowly move down a little bit each day, but the whole system just didn't fit my lifestyle – it wasn't sustainable. There were still those days where I wanted cakes, pizza and other treats. All of the restriction led me to compromise with myself and diet during the week, but then let myself go to town on the weekends. I rationalized that I could always get back on track on Monday.

That in and of itself is an interesting concept: I was reverting back to my old habits of cut, cut, cut and then binge, binge, binge – I was just calling it something else! While dieting during the week and partying on the weekends isn't as extreme, it's so eerily similar and one day I just said to myself "what the heck am I doing." Old habits certainly die hard and I needed more accountability.

Shortly after I found Albany CrossFit, the Paleo diet was the main way of eating that they were preaching at the time and after seeing how fit the CrossFit guys were, I wanted to learn everything about what they did. It went okay for a while, but my issue with living a Paleo lifestyle was that there were so many foods that the diet restricted. I didn't want to be that guy at the party avoiding the cake because it might kill me – that's just not who I am.

I yo-yoed back and forth with Paleo for quite some time, it gave me results, but ultimately I wanted more and I eventually plateaued with that method. One day on Facebook, I saw some success stories Jason had posted along with all this talk about Flexible Eating. He and his clients were getting great results eating donuts and pizza; meanwhile I was sitting at home with my bland grass-fed beef and sweet potatoes. I was envious (and even a little jealous!) of all the fun they were having. I felt like that sick kid trapped at home while all of his friends are outside playing. I had to check this Flexible Eating thing out!

Flexible Eating has opened my eyes to a way of eating that gives me the results I crave and is actually sustainable. Today I am as happy as can be and there are no restraints on how I eat. I feel like I have so much *freedom* with my diet and if my friends want to go out for cheeseburgers and fries, I can actually go with them and not be miserable. I just plan out what I want ahead of time and stick to that plan. It's super simple and I am loving it!

Through Flexible Eating I have also seen a lot of improvements both aesthetically and in my gym performance. I have so much more energy now in workouts and my endurance is the best it's ever been. When it comes to gymnastics movements, there's a fluidity to them now and I'm currently able to perform sixty unbroken pull-ups, a huge increase from my previous max effort of forty. Even my barbell strength has increased – when I previously weighed 205 lbs. and was able to back squat 360 lbs. – but now I am 185 lbs. and squatting 375 lbs. Pound for pound I am a much stronger version of myself!

My advice for others? Stick to it. It's going to be an adjustment at first, but it will become a normal process if you give it some time. Once you start feeling those increases in energy you're not going to want to stop! Also, if you plan ahead there's no doubt you will be successful. Don't leave it until the last second where you have to settle on something. You should never settle when it comes to your health and fitness and, trust me, with Flexible Eating you will never have to.

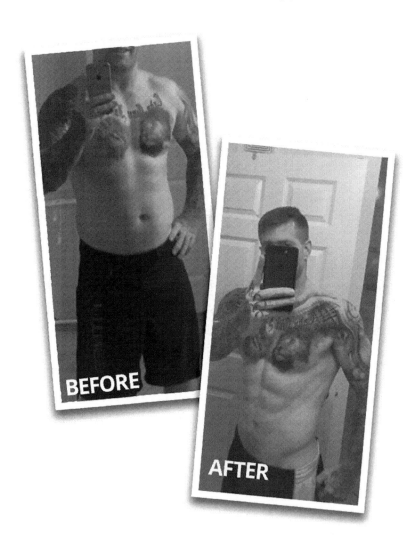

CHAPTER 24

THE SPACE BETWEEN

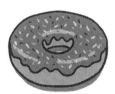

Feeling guilty about eating certain foods (especially the ones you enjoy) is a harmful habit that we have discussed many times. You should never, **EVER** feel bad for eating something. Traditional diets reinforce that guilt by restricting what you eat; successful restriction should never be the goal. Instead, you simply need to be sensible with the amount of food you eat and to remember that at times it is okay to enjoy life and special events because that helps you build and maintain a healthy relationship with food.

Our goal with Flexible Eating has always been to heal this relationship, so that you don't have to turn to food as a coping mechanism.

I know it's easy to get caught up in the hustle and bustle of daily life in the modern world, overlooking problematic and damaging eating habits that may be adversely affecting your emotional and physical health. But at the end of the day we all want the same thing – to live a thriving life. I wholeheartedly believe that Flexible Eating is the best method to lead you down the path toward attaining this.

I have seen how effective Flexible Eating can be in changing my clients both on an aesthetically and athletically adept level, and on a personal, mental one. It's not just about making you look your best; it's about making you feel your best.

The space between you and your relationship with food can be filled by **Flexible Eating**. This flexibility allows you to keep things real and work through challenges that are holding you back from reaching your goals and true happiness. I am one-hundred-percent confident that if you take the messages within this book to heart, and put the information into practice, Flexible Eating will close the gap within your relationship with food and help you truly **OWN YOUR EATING**.

Take a break from reading and give yourself a moment or two to digest what you just read. Use this time to think about your eating habits and current relationship with food.

20   Write a promise letter to yourself. Discuss how your goals, your health, and your life are more important than the food items which may be currently controlling your actions.

_____

_____

_____

_____

_____

_____

_____

_____

21   List and then enact the actions necessary to keep that promise.

_____

_____

_____

_____

_____

_____

_____

_____

_____

This is and always will be about **YOU**. You are worth it; your goals and all of your dreams are worth it too. Be **stubborn** when obstacles are in your way, you really can accomplish a great deal when you set your mind to it.

I hope you have learned some valuable information by completing all twenty chapter exercises, reading the inspirational stories and taking their messages to heart. Now, go use that information, along with what is in this text, to empower yourself to make the changes you desire!

GO OWN YOUR EATING!!

Both Jason & James are passionate about nutrition and Flexible Eating – nothing makes them happier than helping others on their journey. If you need some guidance or assistance they are just a button click away. Please reach out to us by sending an email to Contact@ OwnYourEating.com for Jason or James.AMCD@Yahoo.com to get in touch with James. Visit www.ownyoureating.com for additional support and services they offer – happy eating.

MORE ABOUT THE AUTHORS

JASON ACKERMAN

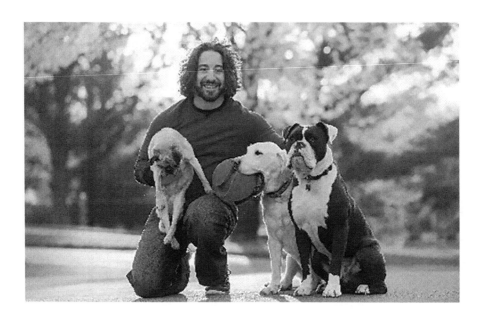

JASON has an extensive health and fitness background, having first entered a gym back in his high-school wrestling days. These trips to the gym at first were meant only to keep him competitive on the mats, but they very quickly became his passion. Within months Jason was interning at his local gym and by 16 years old had his first job as a personal trainer.

Throughout college Jason would work at any gym that would have him. During this time period, Jason honed his craft, spending endless hours watching, reading, and learning everything he could about the fitness industry.

After college Jason continued his journey. He personally trained people, taught fitness classes, managed multiple gyms, and owned his own Yoga Studio.

But it was in 2007 when everything changed…Jason found CrossFit or maybe, CrossFit found Jason. He dove into this new world head first and has never looked back.

Jason was introduced to CrossFit via a friend and an article in Muscle Magazine, like most new CrossFitters he then went home and found everything he could about it online. From there, the rest as they say is history.

Jason started CrossFitting exclusively in his own training and quickly implemented its components in his clients' sessions. Within months Jason attended his first Level 1 seminar and shortly after opened Albany CrossFit.

Jason is currently a CrossFit Level 4 Coach and is also a part of the seminar staff, touring the country instructing at Level 1 & Level 2 seminars. He is very well respected in the realm of CrossFit and was honored to be selected as a judge at the CrossFit Games in 2016.

FOLLOW:

Instagram: @ownyoureating
Website: www.ownyoureating.com

CREDENTIALS:

As well as a Master's Degree in Psychology and 25 years coaching experience in the health & fitness industry, Jason has the following qualifications:

- Precision Nutrition Level 1 Certified
- CrossFit Level 1 Trainer
- CrossFit Level 2 Trainer
- CrossFit Trainer Certification (CF-L3)
- CrossFit Coach Certification (CF-L4)
- CrossFit HQ Trainer
- CrossFit Barbell
- CrossFit Endurance Running
- CrossFit Gymnastics
- CrossFit Kettlebell

- CrossFit Mobility
- CrossFit Nutrition
- CrossFit Rowing
- CrossFit Science
- CrossFit Strongman
- CrossFit Weightlifting

JAMES MCDERMOTT

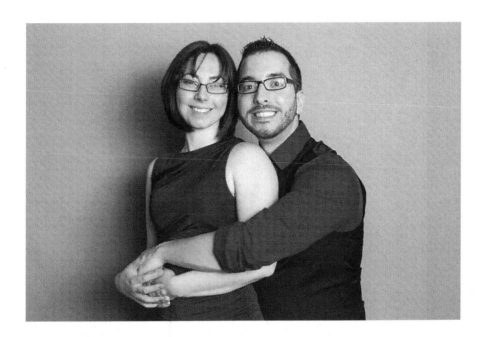

JAMES MCDERMOTT is the Head Coach of Albany CrossFit located in Albany, New York. He specializes in Weightlifting instruction and is an avid competitor in the sport. During his tenure, James has coached several athletes to the podium as well as athletes competing in the CrossFit North East Regionals. While he is very active in sports & fitness now – this was not always the case. As a teenager James struggled with a multitude of health issues as a result of being overweight and living an unhealthy lifestyle. As he matured into young adulthood, James became increasingly unhappy with his life and decided to do something about it. He took responsibility for his personal health and fitness by eating better, exercising and playing sports. Eventually, through a fiery passion for fitness, James began to seek out knowledge on how he could help others live happier, healthier lives.

James entered college with a simple goal: to pursue a career in the fitness industry. He earned a Bachelor of Science in Kinesiology from State University of New York (SUNY) College at Cortland in 2012. His relentless passion to help others led him to discover Albany CrossFit; where he was hired as an intern coach. James dedicated the next few years to Albany CrossFit and saw more responsibility given to him through a series of promotions in the company. He views his role in the gym and the opportunity to help bring about positive change in the lives of others as a privilege. James believes that he truly has the best job in the world. He is always looking for ways he can improve as a coach and expand upon his knowledge to better serve his athletes.

FOLLOW:

Instagram: @jamesamcdermott
Website: www.jamesamcdermott.com

CREDENTIALS:

James' first published book was The Dark Orchestra (Co-Written with weightlifting National Champion Jon North). It can be purchased at www.TheAttitudeNation.com. A few of the certifications James currently holds include, but are not limited to:

- Attitude Nation Level 1 & 2
- Christmas Abbott: The Body Review (Nutrition)
- CrossFit Gymnastics
- CrossFit Endurance
- CrossFit Level 1 & 2 Trainer
- CrossFit Mobility & Movement
- CrossFit Weightlifting Trainer
- Dmitry Klokov Weightlifting Seminar

- Donny Shankle Weightlifting Seminar
- Enderton Strength Online Weightlifting Seminar
- Flexible Eating Seminar with Jason Ackerman
- FuBarbell + The Training Geek: Biomechanical Concepts Applied to Weightlifting
- Glenn Pendlay: Learn To Train
- Jeff Wittmer Weightlifting Seminar
- Jon North & Jared Enderton: Chase The Atmosphere Tour
- Moving With The Maestro: Scapjacked or Jacked-Up Scap?
- New York Weightlifting Academy: Biomechanics of the Jerk
- Original Strength: Pressing Reset – Restoring the Body Through Movement
- Power Monkey Fitness: Gymnastics
- Power Monkey Fitness: Weightlifting (Mike Cerbus)
- Primal Movement Chains – Level 2 – Power Lives In The Transverse Plane
- Punk Rope: Doubles or Nothing Workshop
- Rock Tape: Fascial Movement Taping (FMT) Level 1 & 2
- Rock Tape: Performance Movement Taping (PMT) Level 1
- Rolling on the Floor Laughing: Mobility Workshop
- Tactical Athlete: Kettlebell Workshop with Jeff Martone
- Travis Cooper Weightlifting Seminar
- USA Weightlifting Sports Performance Coach

ACKNOWLEDGEMENTS

FROM JASON:

I could not have done this without my beautiful fiancé and best friend **Roz Glanfield**. No one quite understands me as well as she does. Roz has been patient throughout the hours and hours spent on the phone with James, countless re-writes, interviews with clients, and so much more.

I want to give a big thanks to the *CrossFit* community. From the day that I stumbled upon *CrossFit.com*, my life has never been the same. From founder **Coach Glassman** to every athlete I have had the privilege of coaching, you have all taught me so much. I learn just as much from each of you as I hope you do from me.

Lastly, this would not have been possible without the Own Your Eating Tribe. You all allow me to do what I love on a daily basis and enable me to wake up every morning with purpose. Thank you for supporting me and more importantly trusting me with your health and wellness. It is truly an honor.

FROM JAMES:

"Thank you" is not enough when it comes to showing appreciation for the love and support my beautiful girlfriend **Joanna Toman** gives me on a daily basis. The two of us have been through a lot together and time and time again she shows to be the very definition of patience. When we go on a road trip, she drives so I can work in the car.

When I'm feeling stressed about completing the workload that all of my projects have amounted to she is the one who offers reassuring words to put me at ease. Joanna, I could not do any of this without you. You are my best friend, my partner in crime and the few words typed on this page could never come close to describing how much I love you and how wonderful you truly are.

Also, I would like to thank my family. My mother **Martha McDermott**, father **James McDermott**, brother **Eric Vega**, sisters **Tracy & Anjelica McDermott**, and my grandmother **Marta Vega**. All that I am able to accomplish on my path in life is only made possible because of the bricks laid before me by your collective hands. I dedicate my efforts on this project to the memory of my father James McDermott and grandmother Marta Vega – I wish it were possible for them to read this book – I know they would have enjoyed its contents.

FROM JASON & JAMES TO THE EDITING AND DESIGN TEAM:

One of the key ingredients in regards to the recipe of writing a book is no doubt the creative and editing team that surrounds the project's author(s). That is why we would like to give a special thank you to *The Own Your Eating: The Definitive Guide To Flexible Eating's* editing team: **Joanna Toman, Roz Lytle, Patrick Regan, Roz Ackerman, and Juanita Smart.** These talented individuals took the time to let the meat and potatoes of the text marinate in their minds – asked important questions challenging ideas, made meaningful suggestions, or simply said "that doesn't make sense!" Also, a special thank you to **Victor Marcos.** Victor worked with us to design the front and back cover, all the graphics within the text, and completed the manuscripts typesetting. Victor is an extraordinarily talented artist and we are extremely grateful for his help and guidance. Thank you again to all! We hope that each one of you are as proud of your work on this book as we are.

Made in the USA
Lexington, KY
01 November 2017